Happy Vaginas For The Over 40s

How to resuscitate your ageing asset

and

protect her from menopausal meltdown!

Claire Preston

Illustrated by Vernon Knight

"At 46 one must be a miser; only have time for essentials" Virginia Woolf

Disclaimer

Brand names of products are mentioned in this guide only because they have been recommended by other women who have had good results with them. These brand names do not necessarily represent the best product that will work for you or the full range of effective products currently on the market in your country. You are responsible for your own research and decisions when it comes to treatments and for using products that you purchase over the counter.

Content and illustrations have been reviewed by medical professionals however this guide is not intended to be a substitute for professional medical advice or to be used as a complete source of information about any of the content. It is written as an aid to help you to keep your vagina in the best of health as she continues to mature and to empower you to know when she's crying out for professional attention.

You are solely responsible for the way that you perceive and use this information and you do so at your own risk. You are advised to check with your doctor, specialist or preferred health professional before implementing any of the shared suggestions.

Table of Contents

Table of Contents v

A Quick Word Before You Delve in….. 1

A Look At Your Vaginal 'Map' 2

My Vagina - Not Yours.. 3

The Jewel in Your Vagina –Your Penis on Steroids.................... 4

What Makes My Vagina Unhappy? 5

My Pubic Hair is Thinning and Going Grey.............................. 6

Naked and Sexy – a Pubic Patch Makeover 7

My Vulva is Losing Weight...but I'm Not! 8

Restore a Happy Vulva 9

Not So Happy Vulval Conditions 10

Pamper Your Asset 'down below' 11

Happiness is Not Douching 12

Pelvic Floor Exercises – I Can't be Bothered! 13

Dry Vagina - I Can't Believe It 14

Juice up a Dry Vagina Naturally... 15

Juice Up a Dry Vagina – Other Options 16

Vaginal Tears – Prevention 17

Vaginal Tears – Treatment Options 18

Ouch Sex! – Where To From Here? 19

Slippery Stuff 20

Not So Carefree Slippery Stuff 21

Secretions that Signal a Sad Vagina...................................... 22

How to Test the pH of Your Vagina 23

Natural Vaginal Odor 24

Natural Remedies to Combat Odor... 25

Other Solutions for Vaginal Odor 26

Bacterial Vaginosis (BV) – Bloody Awful................................. 27

Bacterial Vaginosis – Your Home Remedies 28

Bacterial Vaginosis – Reduce Your Risk.................................. 29

BV - What Your Doctor Will Ask You 29

Banish Bacterial Vaginosis 31

Vaginal Thrush – Not Had It? Lucky You! 32

Untreated Thrush Can Holiday Up North! 33

Plumbing Problems.. 34

Reduce Your Risk of a Plumbing Problem 35

Fix Your Plumbing Problems.. 36

Vaginal Bleeding 37

Vaginal Warts = Unhappy Vagina 38

Vaginal Warts - Treatment 39

Sneaky Genital Herpes... 40

Genital Herpes - Symptoms.. 41

Genital Herpes – Prevention and Treatments.......................... 42

How to Live with Herpy the Lodger 43

Chlamydia Alert for the Over 40s.. 44

Prolapses – What Are They? 45

Vaginal Prolapse – Signs and Symptoms................................ 46

Prolapse - Tips to Prevent 47

Vaginal Prolapse - Treatments 48

Electrical Stimulation for a Happy Vagina............................... 49

Designer Vaginas 50

Your G-spot, A-spot AND U-spot - WHAT?!............................. 51

A Happy Vagina Tastes Good 52

Partner Page - Tips for Romeo 53

Sensual Strains for Silly Seniors 54

Spoil Your Way to a Happy Vagina.. 55

A Final Word of Happiness…... 56

Further Sources 57

A Quick Word Before You Delve in...

"After thirty, a body has a mind of its own." Bette Midler

Are you devastated to find that your trusty vagina has started to behave in ways that worry you? The 'old girl' has served you well through passionate nights of lovemaking, probably childbirth and maybe some DIY delights but fallout from the big 'M' (menopause) seems to be taxing her to the max. You've taken her devoted allegiance for granted till now but lately you've noticed that she looks different and just isn't as happy as she used to be.

You haven't quite plucked up the courage to ask your middle aged friends if they are having the same problems. The signs of your vagina's unhappiness are embarrassing, some of them are downright yucky but you suffer in silence, putting off a trip to the doctor till you're desperate and wondering if your lady parts will ever be 'normal' again.

Up top, you're persevering with your anti-wrinkle serums but you've done nothing about 'down there' except maybe notice more grey hairs, debilitating dryness, splits and tears (which hurt like hell) and other distressing symptoms that you're trying in vain to wish away...aagh! Now more than ever ladies, you need to prove to your Yoni, Hoo-Ha, vajayjay, Fru-Fru, toosh, beaver, pussy, lady garden or whatever you call your beautiful vagina, that you LOVE her.

Vaginal Atrophy is enough to scare the bejeebers out of anyone (I can't help but think of things dropping off when I hear the word 'atrophy') but this is a medical term that covers many of the changes and conditions to which we mellow goddesses fall prey as we ripen. Take heart, gorgeous one, you can face these changes full frontal and valiantly resuscitate your 'still breathing pink bits' down below so the two of you can enjoy a long and comfy life together.

As a ripening goddess myself, I gathered this commune of vaginal vagaries as a first stop, self help reference to help you to keep your mellowing vagina happy, to have comfy sex, (but it's your vagina to use, or not, as you wish) a comfy bladder and in the privacy of your own knickers, quickly distinguish between the DIY fixable vaginal worries and the 'must get medical help' ones.

Times have Changed - our generation didn't talk openly about our 'lady parts', let alone about how to keep them happy! You've only got one body and every wee bit of it deserves the best care you can muster so grab a coffee or a glass of your favorite delish, bring your 'flower' into the limelight and let this guide help you to keep your lady garden in full bloom.

Claire Preston

A Look At Your Vaginal 'Map'

To make sure you know which pink parts I'm referring to inside your underwear and what they're called in medicalese (comes in handy for doctor consults) here are two simple drawings showing the external view and the inside side layout of your genitals. If you've never done it, it may be time to drop your drawers and grab a mirror – your faithful vagina will feel your unconditional love!

Your vagina is the *inside* tube (normally 3-5 inches long/7-12cms) the vulva refers to all the outside bits.

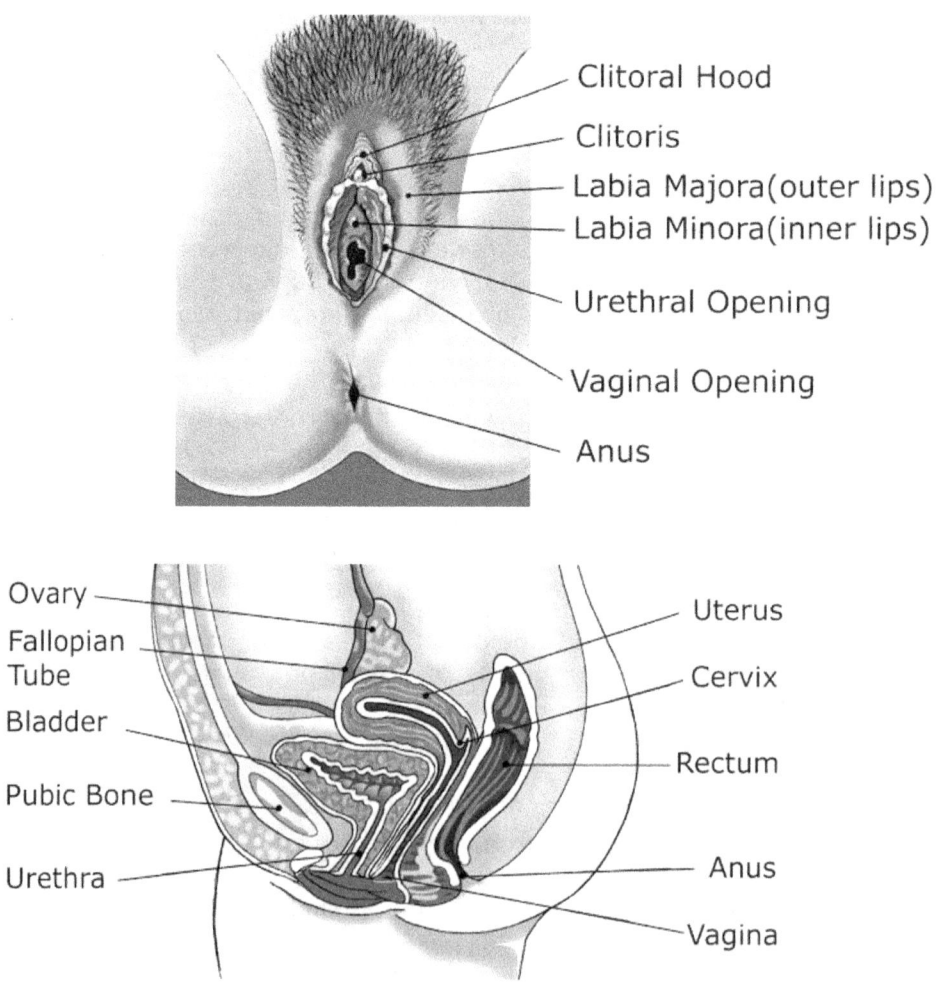

My Vagina - Not Yours

There are many variables when it comes to the health and happiness of your unique vagina. A 'one size fits all' approach does not work, especially in regard to the use of medications, over the counter products and other women's remedies. Sharing solutions to help someone alleviate pain and distress is good, which is what I've done in this guide but please remember...

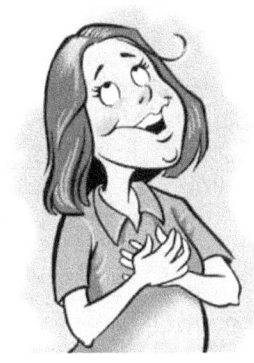

Genetics determine how your body metabolizes everything you put into it and rub on it. Your friend's vagina is different to yours. At this stage in your lives, you can both nourish your assets and expect them to be healthy but don't take them for granted - be sensible and scrutinize everything, remembering that everyone's metabolism and medical background is theirs alone and what works wonderfully well for you may not work as well for your friend. We are good at sharing knowledge, let's do it wisely.

The vaginal health tips and maintenance suggestions in this guide will help you to resuscitate and cheer up your mellowing vagina. 'Pass it forward' if one of these tips or remedies works for you. Share your own successes in vaginal care with your friends and don't be shy in asking for help if you need it. You'll probably find your friends a bit reluctant to raise the subject themselves but relieved that you did, especially if you're all standing on the same dry, uncomfortable and common ground.

Read instructions for vaginal products thoroughly and follow directions faithfully. Before purchasing a new product, check online to see if free samples are available for trial or ask your pharmacist about one. Be vigilant about monitoring results over a period of time when you try a new product so that you can confidently measure how each product performs and quickly counteract any adverse reactions should they occur.

YOU are paying the bill for medical treatments - your vagina has to last you a long time, you have the right to ask as many questions as you need to help you gather information in order to make the right decisions for the future health and comfort of your 'pink bits'. Should you find yourself facing a drastic procedure, such as surgery in your genital area, make sure you shop around for a surgeon with a good track record - just as you would for your car mechanic!

Your vagina is unique – the causes of her woes are shared by millions but the *management* of these is not. Help your vagina to age gracefully by being vigilant, giving her lots of tender, loving care and acting quickly to protect her from everything that negatively affects her health and happiness.

The Jewel in Your Vagina –Your Penis on Steroids

Your clitoris is your erogenous jewel, forming a prime piece of vagina real estate. Let's clear up clitoris confusion. This 'little knob' or 'sex button', which lies under a hood of skin at the top of your vulva, actually has 18 parts, most of them invisible. The little 'nipple', the focus of much sexual delight, is only the tip of a female 'shaft' which extends down to surround the vaginal opening on either side in a sort of inverted 'V', like a pair of legs. In its entirety, your clitoris is almost the same size as the male penis! When little girls ask about their pink bits, serve them well by using the correct words, 'vulva' and 'clitoris' instead of just 'vagina'.

The parts of the clitoris and penis are similar, they are just arranged differently - and the tip, acting like a penis on steroids, is even *more sensitive* than the male's penis glans/tip. Up to about eight weeks of pregnancy, females have the monopoly on fetuses 'generic genitals', all of which appear to be female. When a male fetus begins to produce testosterone, the genitals rearrange to form the penis. The same tissue in the female fetus develops into her clitoris, with the hood equating to the foreskin in men. Brilliant design of the human body eh?

Did you know that your clitoris:

- performs only a sexual job and facilitates multiple orgasms

- has around 8000 nerve endings and is the most sensitive part of your body

- has an 'erection', swells, lengthens and becomes even more sensitive during sex play, responding well to nimble fingers, oral loving and sex toys

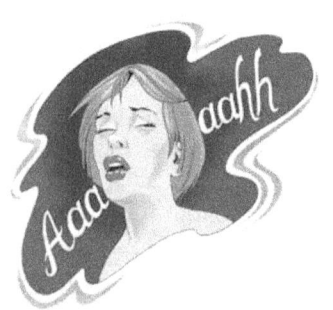

Both the clitoris and the penis work in similar ways to give us orgasms. It's claimed that 2 out of 3 of us need clitoral stimulation to guarantee an orgasm. 'Oohs' and 'Aahs' are more likely to come from sensations from your internal and external clitoris plus your G spot, rather than your vagina itself.

Female ejaculation - yes, some females DO ejaculate (or 'squirt') and it's not from urinary stress incontinence! During an unusually powerful orgasm, glands surrounding the urethral tube can produce an alkaline liquid, similar to seminal fluid that can be ejaculated from the urethral opening. The amount can vary from a few drops to a few tablespoonfuls. Since self lubrication is done by the walls of the vagina, we're not yet sure what purpose female ejaculation serves.

To keep you and your vagina SUPER happy - encourage your sexual partner to be 'clitoris competent' and keep her fit yourself whenever you fancy.

What Makes My Vagina Unhappy?

The big 'M' messing with your hormone factory is a contributing factor in making your vagina sad. The factory just isn't as productive as it used to be in pumping out that estrogen and progesterone. As you've probably discovered by now, your vagina is not the only part of your body affected by a decrease in these two hormones. A drop in your hormone levels could be triggered even sooner if you've misplaced your ovaries. Chemotherapy or radiation on your pelvis and hormonal treatment for breast cancer also impact on the lining of this delicate and sensitive little asset of yours (not to mention menopause meds and life's other bummers).

Vaginal Unhappiness – well done you and take a bow if you're over 40 and don't suffer some form of vaginal unhappiness such as dryness, infection, tears, pain during intercourse, redness, itching, burning or some type of prolapse (God help us). If you've given the slightest nod to any of these saddies, your unhappy vagina is impacting on your quality of life and you owe it to yourself and your 'precious' to do something about it. The tips you'll find in the next few pages will help you to get your vagina smiling again and add that extra boost to your aged care beauty regime.

Your mellowing vaginal tissues, unlike red wine, do not improve with age and despite their valiant efforts to withstand assaults from stress, today's modern diet and man-made lotions and potions, they sometimes have bad 'V' days. Some consistent TLC is needed from now on to protect them from depression due to the painful side effects of thinning, loss of elasticity and loss of lubrication. A swing from slightly acidic to more neutral in your normal vaginal pH balance also makes you fair game for any little entrepreneurial germ seeking a warm holiday resort. If you want to foil Germy's plot to bring along a uterine infection (UTI) for company, examine your vaginal status and action your plan of counter attack.

Your risk of vaginal unhappiness increases once you're over 40 but smoking cigarettes increases it even further (yep, had to let you know). Your vagina needs oxygen to stay in top form. Blood carries oxygen to your vagina via your circulation system and when you smoke you decrease blood flow so you're suffocating the poor girl. Should you ever pop an estrogen therapy pill, it's likely that if you continue to smoke your body will be less responsive and the treatment less effective. Tadah!

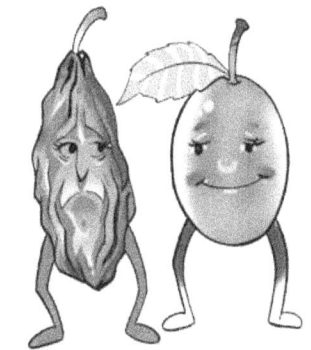

The good news is that in spite of menopause, meds, illness or ageing, you don't have to resign yourself to becoming a sexless, dehydrated prune!

My Pubic Hair is Thinning and Going Grey

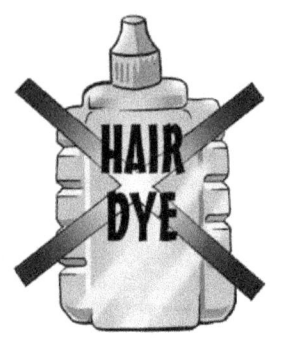

The entrance to your hallowed hallway is sheltered by some thinning thatch so let's start the renovation there and work our way in. A 'Brazilian' wasn't on offer when I was in my 20s but if you're a fan of the totally nude look, wax away Braveheart.

Ageing hair is changing hair, whether it's on your head or on your pubes. We don't deserve it but this is the name of the game when you've clocked up a few decades and Mother Nature has rung the bell for 'The Change'.

Naturally thinning pubic hair reveals more of your vulva which YOU may not like but your partner may *love* so try not to be too dismayed or self conscious about this inevitable change in your pubic coiffeur. Hey, it's more than likely that if you have a male partner, (I'm assuming your non Cougar status here) he's going through the same changes down below *and* he may be losing even more up top as well so chill. Cougars, if Casanova suggests a Brazilian and you're none too keen, you could see how the "I will if you will" reply goes down.

If you're like me, you still rely on your hairdresser and a growing collection of hair products to keep your crowning glory looking great, however, a word of warning if you're tempted to go for a coordinated look a la vulve. This is not a case for a DIY job behind a locked bathroom door with a supermarket special or a liberal application of leftover eyelash tint!

To keep your vulva happy, *don't* do a Charlie Harper with the Grecian 2000 and attempt to dye what's left of your pubic hair yourself. Hair dye chemicals can irritate the delicate skin of your vulva. If you fancy a head to toe matching set or a titillating tint for a special occasion, let a beauty salon professional do it (oh, I couldn't!) and ask for *natural* dyes. You may be surprised at the spice it puts into your love life.

Hair loss due to illness or medication is not a result of normal ageing fall-out - you need to talk to a health care professional if this is the reason for your hair loss. During the discussion remember to also ask about the side effects of your meds on vaginal dryness – you could cop a double whammy here but if you're forewarned, you're forearmed.

A well groomed vulva is a happy vulva, keep her tidy with a regular pubic hair trim if you prefer but always indulge her with some moisturizing (see page 9) - she may be balding but she has her vanity!

Naked and Sexy – a Pubic Patch Makeover

Hairy vulvas are happy vulvas so smile and skip this bit if you are shuddering at the thought of shaving your pubes. Don't let age stop you from styling your thatch though if you fancy a change and you've sufficient hair to style - it can be very attractive to your partner too and your vagina may prefer her new look.

There's nothing medically wrong with removing your pubic hair since your clothes have now taken over the job of protecting your vagina and her mucous membranes. With redundant pubes, an occasional trim of your pubic patch won't do you any harm. Call it good grooming if you like.

Wax away if you wish – I'm just chicken - makes my eyes water just to think about it. If you can't face a professional salon session, here are a few tips for DIY successful shaving:

- a gal's best grooming friend is her Schick Quattro with its narrow head and three adjustable trimmer settings but an electric beard trimmer works well too (he'll never know) DON'T use depilatory creams

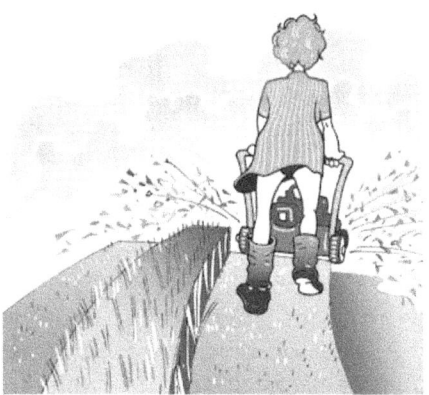

- use a small pair of scissors and a mirror and cut off most of your pubic hair before you shave and shape (wrap hair in a tissue and put in the trash not down the drain)

- substitute *hair conditioner* for shaving cream - a must if you use a disposable razor and want to minimize razor burn, get a close shave and achieve smoothness- this tip WORKS!

- pull the skin tight to help prevent razor burn and use a fresh blade (a tiny dab of rubbing alcohol gets rid of razor burn but ouch!)

- shave downwards in the direction of whatever growth you can find, you will have to work in a few directions to cope with the curves and remove all the hair from sensitive spots

- think carefully about going completely naked as you may end up with painful ingrown hairs and chafing if bare skin rubs against your clothes. A strip or patch style looks neat, is comfortable and you'll soon get used to maintaining it

Have Fun!

My Vulva is Losing Weight...but I'm Not!

...and you're losing hormones too, especially estrogen which has, up until now, kept your plump and juicy vulva in A1 condition. Our vulva is one luscious part of us, apart from maybe our beautiful boobs, where we *don't* want to lose weight.

Your vulva shrinks because the fat deposits and connective tissue under the skin are reduced and no, it's not due to exercise (of any kind). You may also find that you lack the padding you used to have over your pubic bone and that your outer lips (labia majora, check the map) look more pendulous and aren't as plump as they were before (like your boobs?) God bless menopause!

The hood of skin over your clitoris may have shrunk back too so it may look as though this sexy bit has had a growth spurt in its old age, no such luck - this is just one of Momma Nature's wicked illusions.

Make friends with your new genital look - this is normal fall-out from menopausal metamorphosis and part of the graceful ascent into goddesshood. It won't have happened overnight but it may seem that way if you're suddenly scrutinizing parts of yourself that you haven't inspected for a while.

Your vulva is one area where prosthetics and a machine washable toupé would be downright silly and no way am I advocating inflation with any 'plumping stuff' but hey, whatever turns you on. I'm not judging those among you who wish to fill your labia with relocated fat - it's your fat to do with as you wish but please think twice before giving the surgeon the nod. There's a brief explanation of vagina rejuvenation procedures towards the end of this book if you're curious about the queues to go under the knife. Interfering with Nature's 'allsorts' isn't my bag, you don't have to flaunt it to make it feel special anyway, I say.

Your vulva needs some 'aged care' too

Nature won't condone a complete rebirth of this once plump asset but there are a few steps you can take to 'do a Lazarus' in the privacy of your home. I recommend that you use this uniquely feminine weight loss situation as your excuse to invest in some new, mentally anti ageing, sexy lingerie (far more therapeutic than when you were 21 - my friend still wears thongs at 68)

Refocus on essentials ladies - an extra 40 seconds a day is all it takes to indulge your vulva with some delicious restoration. You're never too old to start.

The next page suggests ways in which you can restore a little happiness to your senior vulva.

Restore a Happy Vulva

Surprise and anxiety are common reactions when we discover that ageing has taken its toll on our genitals as well as on our face.

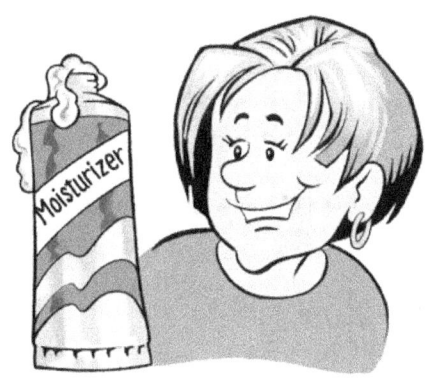

If you have no specific medical concerns, you won't have to overcome any embarrassment in talking to your doctor about this. A happy vulva is a moisturized, succulent vulva. When you give your face its daily drink of moisturizer or dose of collagen, spare a thought for the old girl thirsting down below, your extra gesture of kindness will soon see you both sitting pretty.

External and Vaginal moisturizers - you'll find a range of specially formulated products in most drug stores, I personally prefer the non synthetic products but whichever one you buy, read the instructions carefully and don't be over lavish. A little and often is more beneficial than squirting gobs of the stuff inside you and needing sanitary pads like loofahs to soak up the leakage!

How do external moisturizers work? - moisturizers applied to your external genitals and vulva attract water to the tissue cells to keep them quenched. Most *external* moisturizers are *not* lubricants for *inside* the vagina but they are safe to use on your vulva and surrounding tissues alongside your body moisturizer as part of your daily pampering routine.

- external moisturizers made from plant extracts and natural ingredients include Vulvare or Private Rx External Vaginal Moisturizer

- Yes® is water-based and glycerin free and is currently the only *certified* organic, natural and hormone - free vaginal moisturizer AND lubricant in the world. Yes® doesn't leave any unpleasant residues like some products do and it helps your vagina to keep its acidic balance and protect against Thrush and Bacterial Vaginosis

- a bonus with botanically based restorative creams is that they are usually non staining and non greasy

- if you're prone to yeast infections, avoid products that contain *glycerin*

- avoid petroleum based products as they can harbor bacteria

How to combat vaginal dryness – keep reading.

Not So Happy Vulval Conditions

Is that itch driving you nuts? Itching on your *vulva* is usually due to a skin condition or thrush, not an STD. Get medical help quickly for abnormal conditions on the outside of your vagina. Avoid using soap or over the counter products and if you're in extreme discomfort, toss your knickers girlfriend (shock, horror).

Ingrown hairs – can occur as a result of shaving or waxing, especially if you're a fan of the Brazilian (at my age, you're kidding) - gentle exfoliation helps.

Pimples or cysts – are small hard lumps caused by blocked oil glands in the skin or by ingrown hairs, ignore them unless they hurt, in which case, scoot off to the docs. If you have an itchy vulva, keep your fingernails short and try not to scratch in your sleep (wear cotton gloves?)

Vulval Conditions for which you need specialist help:

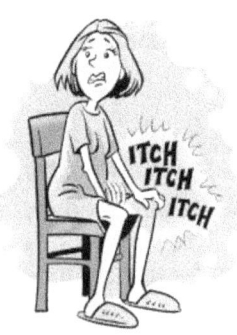

Dermatitis – the itching can be very trying, with red, fluid filled pockets on the skin that break and 'weep'. You can inherit dermatitis or have a reaction to almost anything that touches or irritates your vulva such as toilet paper, laundry detergent, bath products, G- strings, lubricants and so on. Telling you not to scratch is like saying 'Don't worry', but scratching really will make the skin red, stingy and sore and could curb your sex life. Try cool compresses for relief but you really do need to seek help from a doctor to find the best treatment, discover the cause and avoid it in future.

Psoriasis – is a genetic condition which occurs on the hairy skin of the vulva. You may not itch much unless cracks have let in infection. The lesions look salmon pinkish or red but due to the moistness of the vulva, they don't look as scaly as on other areas of the body. Psoriasis is manageable and isn't contagious.

Lichen sclerosus – the skin around your vulva looks pale, dry, shiny, finely wrinkled and may have white patches. This is an extremely itchy condition which is common around menopause. If not treated, scarring and shrinkage of your labia may occur, together with a narrowing of your vaginal opening.

Lichen planus – small lesions can affect your vagina and your vulva and scarring can occur if untreated. A sticky, yellow discharge, soreness, burning, bleeding and painful sex can accompany this condition. There you have it.

Be patient - the skin on your vulva doesn't heal as quickly as skin on other parts of your body so allow more time to treat rashes on this delicate lady part.

Pamper Your Asset 'down below'

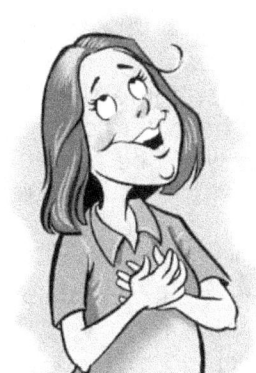

Why should your face have all the fun? When you pamper your face, get into the habit of pampering your other visage too, it's not about getting rid of the wrinkles of course but good servicing keeps the vehicle on the road right? It's more servicing than pampering but I'm assuming the date for your two yearly Pap smear is already on your calendar? Good girl, you're on the ball.

Every goddess should be aware of 'best practice' in aged vaginal care so here 'tis:

Ten tips for pampering your vagina

1. do NOT use strongly perfumed soaps or sprays *inside your vagina* - most body soaps range in pH from 7.0 to 14 so if you prefer to use a soap, find a low pH one made from goat's milk or look for 'natural' soaps at your health food shop (your aim is to keep your vaginal pH between 3-8 to 4.5, when it wants to head towards neutral pH7.0)

2. no douching as a regular hygiene habit - this is one of the biggest causes of vaginal infections and unhappiness, VAGINAS CLEAN THEMSELVES

3. pee when you feel the urge - don't hold it in (we all do this far too often)

4. do your Kegel exercises daily (I know, I know)

5. wear cotton undies to allow moisture to escape and reduce bacterial growth

6. take showers more often than baths

7. wipe from front to back after going to the toilet (read that again)

8. moisturize, moisturize and lubricate, lubricate your vulva and vagina

9. wash your genitals before and after sex - semen is alkaline so it can change the acidic balance of your vagina very quickly once it's in there

10. consider bio identical hormone therapy* or estrogen therapy

Vaginal moisturizers relieve itching, chafing and soreness and help to supply nutrients to those estrogen deprived tissues, 2-3 days application may be enough to regain a comfort level of elasticity but vaginal moisturizers are good to use before sex or as often as you feel you need them.

*Bio identical hormone therapy or estrogen therapy is not usually recommended for breast cancer patients. You should seek a consultation with a medical professional for this treatment.

Happiness is Not Douching

Your vagina will not thank you for douching. As pointed out previously, douching supports infection. Working like a self cleaning oven, your vagina naturally flushes out dead skin cells and excess bacteria. Your vagina is not meant to be sterile and she won't be happy if you upset her pH balance by sacking the hard working little guys (the good bacteria) that Mother Nature put on the job.

Douching only covers up a persistent problem, in some instances, a 'once only' treatment douche, combined with healthy, follow up lifestyle changes may fix a short term vaginal problem but regular douching is a harmful hygiene habit which doesn't rid you of a persistent condition for which you may need medical treatment.

Mucous membranes line your vagina, mouth, nose, eyes and anus and are moist layers of tissue which allow substances to pass through them. Because they do not have the extra protective layer you have on the surface of your outer skin, your mucous membranes are much more easily damaged, irritated and penetrated by 'alien' substances and synthetic chemicals.

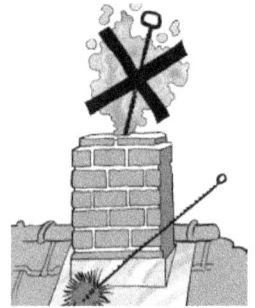 **Your vagina is not a chimney to be swept** so do *not* push any soapy objects up her to clean her, especially strongly perfumed ones. Wash your vulva and if you're soapy in the hold, keep your vagina happy by making sure you rinse her well with lots of water. If you can forego soap altogether so much the better since residue can get trapped in your vagina's comfy little crevices and go 'off', causing an infection. If dryness is her problem, you'll aggravate her further by using bubble baths, soaps and sprays.

Natural vaginal secretions are part of the normal self cleaning process so don't freak out at that smudge in your knickers. I prefer the term 'juices' to 'discharges' - yuk! Let's keep the word 'discharges' for *abnormal* secretions.

Every woman's normal cleansing 'juices' vary slightly - a healthy cleansing juice is clear or whitish and dries pale yellow inside your knickers. Vaginal juice keeps your vagina slippery and the amount you produce will seem less as you exit menopause.

Watch out for any signs that concern you - but don't interfere with the normal functioning of your body. By the time you've finished reading this book, you'll know whether you have a discharge, which is a sign of infection or a healthy juice that is just part of a good self flushing job!

Pelvic Floor Exercises – I Can't be Bothered!

A physically fit vagina is a happy vagina. Yes, I agree it's a pain, especially if you've been born without the exercise gene but if you want a toned vagina, good urinary continence and strong support for your bladder and uterus, you just have to suck it up (literally) and give her an invisible work out at the internal gym. Practice pelvic floor toning or Kegel exercises forever (groan) to keep your vagina smiling.

OK, OK but how do I know if I'm toning the correct bits?

Find the right muscles to work on - pee first then insert your finger into your vagina and squeeze the muscles around it, this is preferable to attempting to stop peeing halfway through. If you've done this well, you will feel your pelvic floor move up and your vagina will tighten. Relax and feel your pelvic floor move down. Don't worry if you don't feel much at first, as you practice, the muscles will strengthen and the tightening will become more evident. Come on, give it a try.

Master your technique (no, you don't have to walk around with your finger up yourself!)

- have a pee to avoid a spill, then sit or lie down. Tighten your pelvic floor muscles and hold for 3 seconds before relaxing for 3 seconds

- repeat this 10 times, that's not so bad eh? Right, now do another 'set' of 10 with 4 second holds this time around. Nah, nah, no breath holding. Don't tighten the muscles in your tummy, buttocks or thighs either, concentrate on tightening the muscles around your vagina and rectum

You'll likely see results in 8-12 weeks (you must be joking!) if you've worked your toning sessions up to 10 second squeezes and done 3 sets of these a day. Attach your 'sets' to a daily job to remind you to do them.

While it's not enough for serious toning, 20 'mini Kegels' while you count to 20 at that red traffic light are better than none at all. If you pull up next to another goddess at the lights and she's tight lipped you'll know what she's up to.

By the way, Kegels are great for men too - they can contract their muscles to delay ejaculation!

Dry Vagina - I Can't Believe It

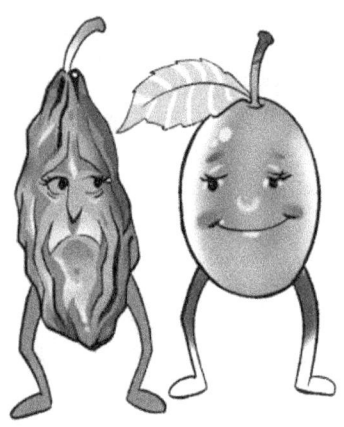

One moment all seems fine, then the next time you have a love session with your partner, ouch, it brings tears to your eyes and a tear in your tender region or a burning sensation that's sore for days. You aren't imagining this and you haven't failed at Pilates. 20 million women in the US suffer from vaginal dryness which doesn't sound like a big deal but boy, can it rain on our parade - if we let it.

"Use it or lose it!" Well you would if you could, right? Are you sick of hearing this as a drought remedy for your dehydrated tissues? Dryness needs conquering, regardless of what type of sexual future lies ahead for you. Dryness can lead to tiny cracks in the walls of your vagina which increase your risk of infection. Regular sex may cultivate your lady garden but the ground needs good preparation first.

That damned drop in your estrogen levels is a major contributor to the drought conditions in your lady garden but if you can accept that this process is all part of Big Momma's natural ageing plan for most goddesses your age, your indomitable attitude will make the problem less traumatic and you'll be able to launch your recovery charge.

Stress, stress and stress! Adjusting to your changing body, coping with a full time job, ageing parents, grandchildren, housework, shopping and generally being superwoman seven days a week, clocks up mileage on your stressometer. Top these stressors off with medications you may be taking and no wonder your poor little vagina is sulking, she was looking forward to a fun filled, indulgent retirement. Well, it's never too late to establish the vagina superannuation fund.

Vaginal dryness is in the 'top ten' list of popular symptoms for the over 40's goddess and can be worrisome to deal with, especially if you're still determined to have a healthy sex life but don't want to become an HRT junkie. Be proactive. There are several ways to make your vagina smile again, she may be a delicate flower but she's resilient and responds well to pampering!

Warning: Common problems caused by a dry vagina and what to do about them are identified next but remember, where estrogen therapy may be the way to a happier vagina for many, it is *not* usually recommended for anyone with a history of breast cancer.

Juice up a Dry Vagina Naturally

A juicy vagina is a happy vagina. These natural remedies have hydrated other thirsty vaginas – maybe one of them could work for yours?

Natural remedies:

- guzzle lots of water – 8 pints a day will flush toxins away and really help to moisturize your vagina - but we just don't do it do we?

- hemp seed oil – "*An edible oil with superior nutritional and therapeutic properties*".Dr. Andrew Weil - make sure it is nitrogen flushed, cold pressed and in a dark bottle (not the dodgy stuff from China)

- insert a Vit E capsule into your vagina - Vit E oil can also be applied externally to be absorbed internally to nourish dry tissue (can be sticky)

- try a raw food diet and add healthy fats from nuts, linseed and avocado

- chamomile, ginseng, calendula and black cohosh soothe inflamed tissue

- sesame oil - massage the walls of your vagina every day for at least 7 days with a cotton pad dipped in the oil

- olive oil*, coconut oil and Crisco oil can be used but not if you're using condoms

- put one glass of water into a pan, add 1 tsp fenugreek seeds, boil for 15 minutes, allow to cool and drink it once a day

- make a thin broth from boiling a small handful of rice in two cups/500 ml of water and drink as often as you like

- practise whatever 'turns you on' for at least 20 mins before intercourse, mmm, sounds better than rice broth and also sends an SMS to your brain to increase output of disease fighting enzymes/vaginal juices

- make sure your partner adds to your wetness during oral sex, if you get my dribble

- avoid relying on mineral oil and petroleum jelly – these upset the balance of your vaginal juices, can breed bacteria and have a detrimental effect on latex condoms

*Bacteria can grow in olive oil and can also be trapped by residue left behind by other lubricants and oils if you don't wash them off after use.

Juice Up a Dry Vagina – Other Options

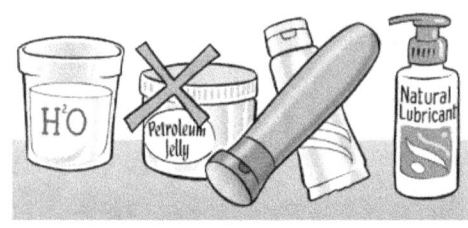

A dry vagina is an unhappy vagina; she feels tight and is easily damaged so you need to *coax* her into juiciness. You don't need to go overboard with sticky creams or grease her up like an axle. Juicing up with the aid of lubricants makes for comfy sex (either solitary or shared) and nowadays is a must for lusciousness in your lady garden.

To promote juiciness:

- Replens – estrogen free, contains a special molecule that draws water into vaginal tissue - use daily for about a week, then two to three times a week as needed

- Yes®, Pjur For Women, KY LiquiBeads, O'My, Vagifem

- Crisco shortening(some women swear by this) or soy vaginal cream

- Bio Indentical Hormones* – are chemically processed from sarsaparilla, Mexican yam or soy bean and are so named because the molecules in them are identical to those in your body. Available in many forms including capsules, topical creams and gels, consult a professional to find out your exact dosage

- natural progesterone supplements♥ help to balance hormone levels and neutralize the dangers of excess estrogen

- Estriol cream and steroid creams may be recommended by your doctor if you don't have a history of breast cancer. Natural estriol creams* can be bought over the counter, synthetic estriol creams are the ones often prescribed by a doctor

Regardless of which remedy works for you, please try to get down those 8-10 glasses of water a day and if a daily exercise routine isn't your thing, try to be active in some other way to keep the circulation in your nether regions throbbing.

*Bio Indentical Hormones are becoming popular as 'natural' products are more sought out these days, however, controversy still reigns around whether they are any more effective than synthetically manufactured hormones. Not all Bio Identical Hormones are FDA approved.

♥A saliva test can reveal your hormone levels so that the dosage can be tailored to suit your particular needs but there is some question as to whether or not this test accurately reflects the hormone levels in your blood or corresponds to menopause symptoms.

Vaginal Tears – Prevention

It's sheer hell if the fragile skin around the opening of your vagina tears every time you push something past it, intercourse is a nightmare and sympathetic murmurings from your doctor don't help. When you have a tear, your clothing rubs and it hurts even when you wipe your bum (wet, folded, lint free toilet paper helps). You need a plan of action to prevent tears happening in the first place.

If you already have a tear or split, you need to allow Mother Nature to heal it up, *undisturbed* if possible, which it often does with cream and TLC (see next page) then 'train' the tissues around your vagina to become stronger and more flexible:

- do daily perineal massage- sit or lie down, relax, then use your oiled thumb inserted gently, to massage around the vaginal opening, pushing gently forwards to stretch the area that's weak (Vit E cream, Calendula ointment or heavy white zinc based baby cream are also good)

- avoid anything that might give you an allergic reaction near your vagina such as colored or perfumed toilet paper, talc, vaginal or hemorrhoid creams, latex condoms, glycerin, petroleum jelly

- use estriol cream or estriol pessaries to help thicken the vaginal tissues and reduce the risk of tearing

- use a vibrator and water based lubricant to gently stretch the skin around the vaginal opening and to get your vagina used to the exercise, especially if there's been a long spell between 'visitors'

- gently stretch your vagina with a dildo or a candle using a slow circular motion (yes, recommended by a gyno to stretch tissues) and use a pH balanced, water based lube

- go slowly during intercourse and keep yourself well lubricated - it's almost a reflex action to tense up in anticipation of tearing but consciously relax as much as possible and take your time - guide your partner to 'resting' at the door a while before entry

- ask your doctor about cortisone ointment which is the only solution for some poor darlings who tear frequently

- intercourse isn't the only way to have enjoyable or satisfying sex – foreplay and using fingers to slowly arouse the body helps your vagina to become naturally moist and if the poor old girl isn't responding, help her along with some lube

N. B. Get checked by your doctor if vaginal tears persist.

Vaginal Tears – Treatment Options

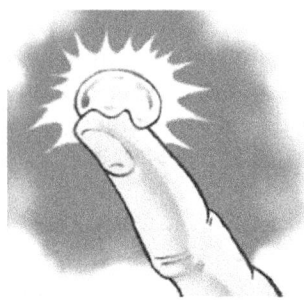

Suffering from constant pain in or around your vagina can lead to mental agony as well as physical discomfort, especially if you are sexually active. It's no consolation I know but tearing around the vagina happens to sexually athletic *young* women too, not just to us menopausal ladies. This doesn't mean that your days as a sexual being are numbered or over. Untreated wounds can become infected so please persevere in your search for a solution.

Unless you solve the dryness issue, you're likely to keep getting tears and possibly creating inelastic scar tissue so having sex or a pee becomes a pain instead of a pleasure. Once you find a solution, you'll be able to regulate how often you need to use it as part of your ongoing vaginal maintenance plan. Think reclamation and resuscitation ladies, you and your precious lady parts deserve it.

After a consultation with a doctor or gynecologist one of these options may be offered to you:

- estrogen cream - topical creams are often more effective than popping a pill and less estrogen enters your blood stream and liver this way but don't over apply. Using an applicator, you insert the cream into your vagina where it gradually helps to 'thicken' the surrounding tissues

- estrogen tablet or pessary – an alternative to cream, quick to insert and great for the traveler (not so messy, use at night while you're horizontal to avoid dribbling)

- oral estrogen – ask your doctor about the connection of this to gall bladder disease if you're post menopausal. Oral estrogen can also lower testosterone so if your libido is fading you may make things worse here

- estrogen ring – a flexible plastic ring which is inserted into the upper part of your vagina and which releases about 3 months steady supply of estrogen and it doesn't interfere with intercourse

- Cetaphil and Eucerin lotion - as preferred by some women, are recommended by dermatologists and won't burn or clog your skin

- surgery – an absolute last resort for the treatment of tears and not one to be taken without lots of investigation and questions to your specialist (I'd also be asking someone who's already 'been there, done that')

Keep some lubricant and/or vaginal moisturizer on call as backup.

Ouch Sex! – Where To From Here?

Maybe it's been a while since your vagina has had a visitor so you may feel anxious as to how it will go when you next get lucky. Cheer up, help is at hand if you're willing to step out of your comfort zone for a little vagina 'retraining'.

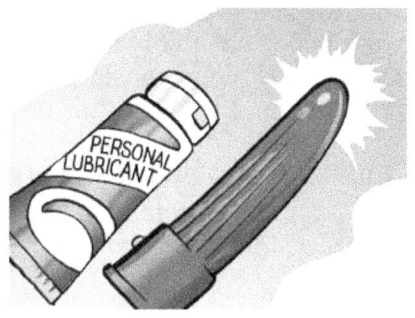

A babe can *sail* down a vagina during childbirth so a decent sized penis should have no problem right? Well, technically that may be true but unless you're relaxed, properly aroused and *lubricated*, intercourse over 40 can be nothing like those Warner Bros. scenes.

Anxiety doesn't help - the more you worry, the worse it gets. 'At our age' it's very important to make sure that sex is something that you want, if you're not in the mood, you won't be relaxed and there's a greater chance of a wince rather than a whoohoo! Creativity and sensitivity in the love arena are definitely assets.

Ok, you're 'up for it' but you need a bit of help with the program:

- grab lots of water-based lube - for your partner as well as yourself

- 'train' at room temperature where you are relaxed and warm enough

- play slow, soothing music to accompany your exercises (see page 54)

- make your own set of personally sized 'training' dilators, increasing in sizes, from vegetables like carrots, zucchinis and cucumbers (peel to size) – warm them in hot water, put a condom over each and slather lube on and around your vagina: wiggle your tool of choice gently to help stretch the vaginal opening

- employ a sex toy for 'temp work' to gradually expand your vagina - feel queasy? Think of it as a medical aid!

- allow plenty of warm up time before intercourse, a little experimenting can spice up graying ardor and a sense of humor goes a long way to relaxing your partner into the role of love guru/personal trainer. If you've previously had vaginal tears, get your partner to 'rest at the door' for a minute before pushing inside

- sit on-top during sex for more control and guidance (if your arthritic knees permit!) or lie on your side to decrease the depth of penetration

"For me, love is very deep but sex only has to go a few inches"...Stacy Nelkin

Slippery Stuff

Once you've gracefully accepted a little help for 'happy hour', do your homework when choosing a commercial lubricant as they are not all equal. Your vagina will benefit from your considerate and caring efforts to protect her from menopausal meltdown and she'll do her best to reciprocate when she's centre stage.

Some natural lubes with which to moisturize your vagina include olive oil, Vitamin E oil, acidophilus and comfrey ointment. As I've mentioned already, bacteria can grow in left over lube 'residue' and olive oil so clean up carefully and be vigilant.

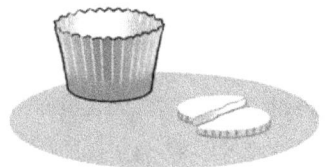

A tip to avoid interrupting the moment: 'prepare something earlier' by putting a tspn. of liquid coconut oil into a silicone cupcake cup and freezing it. Before play commences, insert half a disc into your vagina before you light the candles and slip into something sexy.

An ideal lube should:

- be easy to apply

- stay 'slick' but not feel sticky, even in the afterglow

- not dry up quickly or leave you feeling dry

- not irritate you or your partner

- not taste bad (I have to cover all bases right?)

- feel smooth and silky, like your vagina's natural lubrication

Water based lubes are PH balanced and will make your dry vagina very happy because they will soak into your delicate vaginal tissue, keep it moisturized and protect it from splits and tears. Sweet! Reapply as you need, these are safe if swallowed.

If you are prone to yeast or bacterial infections find a lube *without* glycerin - such as Yes®, Astroglide Natural, Sliquid brand lubricants, Slippery Stuff, Liquid Silk, Maximus, and Hathor Aphrodesia.

Silicone lubes - if you're flying solo with a sex toy and you don't want it to melt, don't use a silicone based lube. Silicone lube is glycerin free but is best kept for water play, it's also great for doing self breast exams in the shower because it gives a nice gliding effect and won't rinse off with just water.

Not So Carefree Slippery Stuff

If you are plagued by yeast infections, yet still delight in sumptuous sex romps with chocolate syrup and whipped cream, you need to listen up. If you want to avoid fuelling a 'yeast fest', save that syrup for your banana split. There are 3 big NO, NO's to heed when it comes to 'slithering up' your vagina:

1. Avoid anything that contains sugar (supports yeast growth)

2. Avoid using a lube that contains petroleum oil (dissolves rubber/latex and can trap bacteria longer because it's sticky)

3. Avoid using a lube that contains glycerin (sugar again)

Fact: Post menopausal women are more susceptible to allergic reactions from chemicals in lubes. Here's a quick word about *parabens*, which along with sugars/glycerin and petroleum in lubes are also included on my own 'no, no' list.

Parabens are preservatives which are used extensively in cosmetics and are also found in lubricants. We still do not know enough about the effects of long term exposure to parabens. One small research study has detected parabens in breast tumors and now questions a link to this type of cancer - another study suggests that parabens may actually accelerate skin ageing.

If you react badly to parabens, check the ingredients list on the lube pack carefully or play safe with Astroglide Free which is free of parabens. I mention this lube first because it is usually fine for women who can't tolerate other lubes.

Paraben free water based lubricants include: Sliquid, Hathor and O'My. KY jelly is a water-based lubricant and popular with many but check the label for a product without parabens *and glycerin* if you're inclined to favor yeast infections. Sylk is paraben free but contains grapefruit seed extract (GSE) which causes a burning feeling in those who react to this particular ingredient.

Most silicone based lubricants, like Eros and Platinum, do not contain parabens, are not absorbed into your skin and usually do not contain anything that will cause an allergic reaction, they are also harmless if swallowed but taste yucky. Silicone lubes are not compatible with latex or 'cyber skin' sex toys.

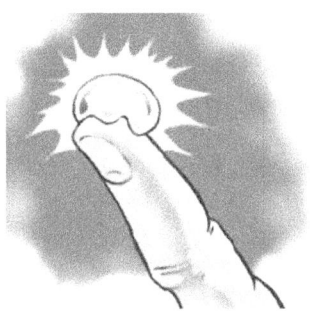

Bottom line (pardon the pun) Find a lube that *likes you* and stick to it.

Secretions that Signal a Sad Vagina

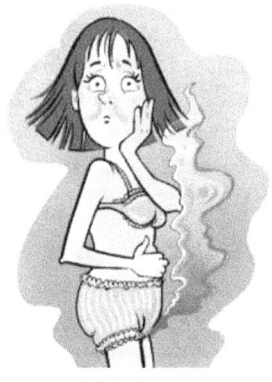

We're talking *discharges* here ladies, not natural juices. Let's be honest, unless you're a regular sufferer, who among us doesn't feel the teeniest bit uncomfortable discussing a vaginal discharge? Every day millions of women have to overcome their embarrassment to front up to a doctor with this problem………. you can too.

'Happy' vaginal juices are pH balanced and *slightly acidic*. After menopause, your vaginal juice tends to lose its pH balance and wobble towards pH neutral. If you notice a change in your vaginal juice (which occurs with a pH wobble) a vaginal pH test kit will confirm if you need some balancing assistance. Normal juices can differ between friends. You know your own juice better than anyone so keep your senses finely tuned and pay attention when you pull down your knickers.

When your vagina sends you these signals seek medical advice sooner rather than later:

- strong or unpleasant odor

- a lot of watery discharge

- painful and frequent peeing

- a discharge that contains blood

- a thick, yeasty discharge that has small curds like cottage cheese in it

- a discharge accompanied by pain in your pelvic area

- any other discharge that causes you burning or itching

- a discharge that is greenish, grayish, *strange* yellowish or pinkish (well, that just about covers the full palette!)

- feeling like you to want to pee even though you're empty

A vaginal pH test kit is available over the counter or online if you'd rather go down the DIY path first to find out if you might have an infection.

How to Test the pH of Your Vagina

A vagina with a normal pH is a happy vagina – one with an 'upset tummy' isn't. A change in the balance of your vagina's acidic juices requires you to settle her down and bring her back to normal again as soon as possible. A dose of Gaviscon just won't cut it.

If your vagina is exuding a different odor or her secretions have changed, you need to find out if she has an infection. If you experience itching or burning when you pee and want to confirm the status quo before you go to your doctor, you can test the pH of your vagina with a DIY test kit bought over the counter. These kits are almost identical to the ones used by doctors and while you may need some extra lab tests for a proper diagnosis, they are good for a DIY job.

What is a vaginal pH test anyway?

It is a simple test that shows you the *acidity* level of your vaginal juice. A pH scale ranges from 0-14 so a pH reading of 7 is neutral (like distilled water). A pH reading lower than 7 shows that a solution is acidic, whereas a reading of, say, 11 would show that a solution is more basic or alkaline (like household detergents)

A Normal Vaginal pH reading is 3.8 - 4.5

Each pH test kit will come with its own set of instructions but basically you hold the special strip of paper supplied in the kit against the wall of your vagina for 5 seconds. After a few minutes a color appears which you then match to a color chart supplied. The chart will show you the corresponding pH reading for your vaginal secretion.

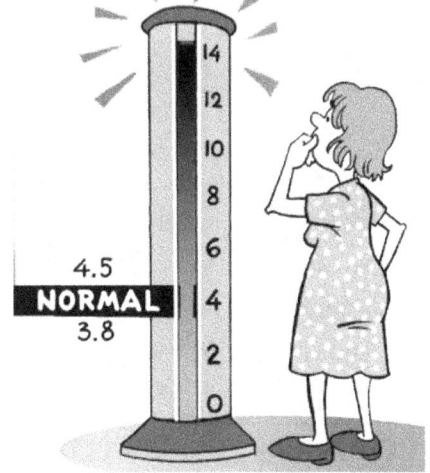

If your pH reading is BELOW 3.8 it's likely that you have a yeast infection, to confirm this yourself (you've guessed it) you can buy an over the counter yeast infection kit or see a doctor for confirmation and treatment.

If your pH reading is OVER 4.5 (sign of vaginal atrophy and loss of acidic balance) you really should toddle off to get checked for an infection like *bacterial vaginosis* (BV) or some other little lodger. A change in your vaginal pH doesn't always indicate an infection but these test kits are pretty reliable.

Natural Vaginal Odor

A happy, well balanced vagina has a healthy, inoffensive smell, *regardless of her age*. You're likely to notice a change in your vaginal aroma when your vaginal pH status alters. Actually, it's not so much your vagina that smells but the juices she secretes. Who among us hasn't ever worried about the cleanliness of our vagina or if she has an off putting pong which others can smell like BO or bad breath?

Your vagina has a happy little family of bacteria called 'vaginal flora', (mainly Lactobacillus) which live on the walls of your vagina doing a great housecleaning job. The good guys strive to stop other more harmful bacteria from taking over and upsetting the status quo, predisposing you to infection and odor.

The balance of bacteria and yeast varies from vagina to vagina which means that each vagina will have its own cleansing 'juice' and unique aroma. A healthy secretion is clear or whitish and dries a pale yellow inside your knickers.

Bacteria, parasites and yeast cells inside your vagina produce waste matter and byproducts that can buildup to give off an unpleasant whiff. You may notice you smell slightly stronger at the end of the day.

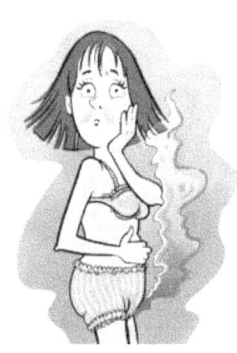

If you naturally have a strong aromatic 'presence' but you don't have an infection like bacterial vaginosis, be really conscientious about washing your genitals every day especially in Summer when we all perspire more. Excessive vaginal sweating allows bacteria to multiply and cause odor.

Please resist the urge to douche or to use perfumed soap, sprays or feminine washes, as all of these are harmful to a healthy and very sensitive vagina. Chemical products inside your vagina can cause an over production of bacteria, especially now that your internal environment is less acidic.

Regular douching can irritate your delicate vulva and lead to infections that cause an offensive pong. Chemicals can also get into your urinary tract through your vagina and cause an uncomfortable urinary tract infection (UTI).

The smell of your body is sensual – if your lover relishes your warm aroma, make the most of it but be ready, if the need should arise, for a little diplomacy.

If your smell is really disgusting it's likely that you have some type of infection so it's a doctor's visit for you. Far better to know the cause and get rid of it than to be anxious about sex and risk embarrassing looks from those close by.

Natural Remedies to Combat Odor

If you naturally have a strong aromatic 'presence' (as in stinky) which is not due to an infection, *over washing* of *your vagina is not the answer*.

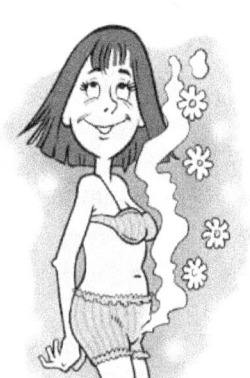

These remedies come recommended by other freshly fragrant women:

- eat more fruit and celery

- eat more natural, unsweetened yoghurt

- cut out or cut down on your intake of bread, mushrooms, sugary foods, beer and coffee (I'm afraid so) which can increase the amount of yeast in your vagina

- mix 2 *drops* of tea tree essential oil in 6oz of purified water and apply around your vaginal area. Tea tree oil is antifungal/ antibacterial but do *not* use it undiluted, *ouch*, it may burn (test a patch first on inner thigh)

- add 1 TBSPN. liquid chlorophyll to 8oz. of water and drink this twice a day. Chlorophyll is an internal deodorizer. Don't panic if your pee or poo looks green or if your tongue looks black, these are normal effects (I'm not sure I could handle the comments about a black tongue though)

- dip a tampon into natural, *unsweetened* yoghurt and insert into your vagina for an hour or two. The healthy bacteria in the yoghurt will help to fight any unhealthy bacteria. Thoroughly rinse your vagina after removal of the tampon (check with your doctor before trying this one)

- ditch the leggings and lycra bike shorts (sweat + bacteria = pong)

- you may have to rely on cotton undies, pantiliners and loose clothing for good ventilation of your nether regions to get you through the day

- pee after sex to flush out semen and bacteria – sperm can hang around for several days and affect the odor of your vagina

- smegma is a normal secretion of your sebaceous (oil) glands that mixes with dead skin cells and can collect under the hood of your clitoris so if you see this whitish, cheese like substance just wash it off

Your partner may get used to your natural smell, pleasure you in a different way or deal with your strong 'essence' by dabbing a little something under their nose before sex! Importantly, discuss how you both feel about it so that you can tackle the issue together.

Other Solutions for Vaginal Odor

Here are some other solutions that women have found effective in neutralizing external odor causing bacteria around their vaginas. These suggestions go against my preference for not meddling with Mother Nature but given that they contain a high proportion of natural minerals and don't seem to cause any allergic or adverse reactions with their fans, I thought it only fair to pass them on.

For external use only, do not use inside your vulva or vagina:

- Bionsen – an aluminum and paraben free 'anti- odorant' rather than a deodorant. Made from Japanese mineral crystals to which you add water in a spray bottle - refills up to 5 times and does not block sweat glands or irritate sensitive skin. Shower Gel is available too

- Pit Rok – a paraben free crystal deodorant containing natural mineral salts that suppresses bacterial growth yet is kind to skin. The spray contains aloe vera and calendula for skin conditioning

- Femanol- a natural herb supplement which contains herbs, zinc, biotin, neem bark extract (antifungal/antibacterial and destroys odor causing bacteria) Vitamin B, selenium and deodorized garlic (natural antibiotic)

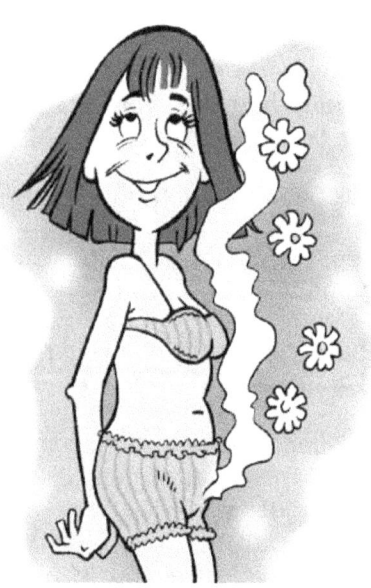

Synthetic clothing holds moisture in which odor-causing bacteria thrive, which is why it's best to opt for cotton fibers where possible With a wide range of attractive cotton undies on the shelves nowadays, you don't have to settle for Bridget Jones knickers unless you're a comfort before elegance devotee.

If your strong odor gets worse or persistently defies your self-help attempts to subdue it, perform a vaginal pH test then get checked for an infection by a health professional (this is mandatory if you also have an offensive discharge and/or urinary problems). It's easier said than done but try to reduce your stress if you have this problem, your vagina will thank you.

Bacterial Vaginosis (BV) – Bloody Awful

That happy little family of bacteria who live in your vagina do a great balancing job, going about their cleaning business and normally not causing you any problems. However, if something causes the acidic balance in your vagina to change, marauding bacteria will take over and you'll have one unhappy vagina who will make her misery felt and might even muscle in on your sex life.

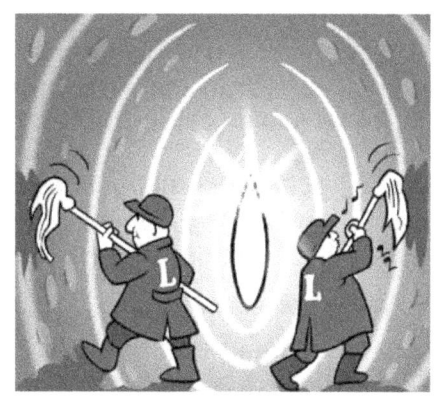

The resident good guy bacteria in your vagina are lactobacilli, the same bacteria found in yogurt (dubious claim to fame).

Bacterial Vaginosis is a common infection - it only affects women (whoopidoo) and you'll be one of the lucky ones if you never get it. It's a bummer if you get it frequently but persevere till you find something that works for you, you can get rid of it. BV is not an STI but sexual activity can exacerbate it, neither is it a yeast infection like thrush which we'll look at next.

What causes bacterial vaginosis? No one is absolutely sure. A change in your vaginal pH (surprise!) causes the mischievous, gate crashing bacteria to party on and multiply. More baddies than goodies in your vagina result in inflammation and infection. A reading over 4.5 on a vaginal pH test scale can be a sign that you have BV. Aside from vaginal atrophy, your risk of BV increases if you have multiple sex partners, have oral sex, if you regularly douche and if you are suffering from stress.

Symptoms of BV: bad news is that you can have it without these symptoms:

- a clear or colored (milky, grey or white) discharge from your vagina that may be light or heavy

- a strong smell that may be fishy, especially after intercourse

- itching and redness

- burning when you pee

Don't ignore BV just because it's a mild infection. Untreated, a chronic infection may get up into your uterus or fallopian tubes (if you still have an intact set). It's not usual for a male partner to need any treatment (some perk!) but a female partner may. If you have a vaginal pH reading over 4.5 you have two options, try a DIY remedy first or make an appointment to see your doctor.

Bacterial Vaginosis – Your Home Remedies

Bacterial vaginosis is a recurring nightmare for lots of women. To banish it, you need to kill the bad bacteria in your vagina, restore the acidic balance, get the good guys back in there again then work out what upset your lady garden in the first place so you can prevent a recurrence in the future. Easy peasey, yeay, right.

Not all remedies will work for everybody because our bodies are so different but these women to women tips, shared by women who are fed up with repeat courses of antibiotics that don't work, are alternatives you may wish to consider:

- kill the baddies with a douche (oh no!) of 3% hydrogen peroxide diluted ½ and ½ with water if too strong Use a medicine syringe, rinse twice

- grapefruit seed extract douche, 10-20 drops diluted in 2 cups of water

- at night, re-introduce the good bacteria with some live lactobacillus acidophilus. Syringe up 2 tspns of the liquid culture or soak a tampon with it and insert. TIP: use a *small* tampon in a *large* applicator tube to insert a soaked tampon into your vagina. NB. There is no strong, documented evidence that this actually helps in treating BV but it's claimed to be successful by some - ask your doc if you want to try it out

- a *mild* vinegar solution douche for a 'one off' remedy has worked for some but be warned - you may end up encouraging yeast cells to thrive

- the FAC oral cocktail – 1000mg folic acid a day plus 2 acidophilus pills a day helps to support the friendly bugs in their cleaning job downstairs

- 2000 IU Vit D3 per day

- a glass of buttermilk per day and cut out sugars and carbs from your diet

- 4 oz unsweetened cranberry juice twice a day

- if you've got one, make your Romeo wash his pink bits thoroughly to support the cause!

- use a pH test kit to see which way you're secretions swing

If you have recurring bouts of BV – it means that you still haven't found out what is throwing your pH balance out of whack and *this is the real secret* to getting rid of this pesky nuisance for good. Perseverance will win out my friend so give it your best shot.

Bacterial Vaginosis – Reduce Your Risk

Given that even the experts do not fully understand the exact causes of bacterial vaginosis, the best thing you can do to reduce your chance of getting a bout of BV is to avoid upsetting the delicate natural pH balance of your vagina (you must have got this by now). It's difficult to prevent something from happening if you don't know what triggers an occurrence in the first place.

Green lights for reducing risk of BV:

- wash your genitals once a day - no antiseptics, no use of scented, non fatted soaps on your vagina, if you must use soap, Dove and Neutrogena make a super-fatted soap with added oils that are low in alkalis (remember your vaginal secretions need to be kept slightly *acidic*)

- do NOT douche (as a regular hygiene method rather than a one off treatment for BV)

- Echinea, Garlic, and Vitamin C will help fight off infection and keep it away if you continue to take them

- use *mild* detergents to wash your underwear

- reduce your number of lovers (quality rather than quantity, right?)

- use a condom and lots of lube, especially if you're planning to have multiple sex partners

- make sure that any sex toys you use are really clean before using in your vagina (if you get my drift)

- check with your doctor before trying any products or practices that a new partner may suggest to you but which seem dubious

- pull the plug on intercourse - I know, I know but this suits some post menopausal women very well and there are still many other ways of having satisfying sex. By the way, BV is seldom found in women who have never had sexual intercourse

N.B. your vaginal health is directly linked to your overall health and a strong immune system. Bugs are opportunistic little pests that LOVE weakened immune environments so look after your own well being.

BV - What Your Doctor Will Ask You

You and I could teach some male doctors a thing or two when it comes to bedside manners especially when we are seeking refuge from the big 'M' fall out. We expect and deserve SO much more than a prescription. We need all the empathy we can get to talk about our intimate problems with someone else. A 6 minute consult doesn't give us the time we want to express how we feel about changes in our lady parts. In the face of reality and the consultant's clock, make the most of the consult session by doing a bit of pre appointment preparation:

Be well prepared – take with you a list of any home remedies or over the counter treatments you've tried, even if you've had no success with them and be prepared to answer some intimate questions about your sex life and hygiene habits. Don't accept derogatory comments regarding your DIY attempts to get rid of your BV and make sure your doctor realizes how BV is affecting your daily life.

"I'd like to be checked for a vaginal infection" should get you off to a good start if you're sheepish about describing nasties in your nether region. Let the doc ask the questions and don't wear a tampon or douche for at least 24 hours before your appointment. You'll likely be given a pelvic examination during which a swab will be taken of your vagina and sent for testing in a laboratory.

Here are examples of some questions your doctor might ask you:

- what symptoms do you have?

- how long have you had these symptoms?

- are you sexually active? (you may have to elaborate)

- how do these symptoms impact on your sexual activity?

- do you use a douche or feminine vaginal spray?

- do you take bubble baths or use scented soaps?

- what current medications and/or vitamins or over the counter supplements are you taking?

- what have you tried so far to get rid of the symptoms yourself?

Vaginal discharges in menopause are very common. While this condition may be a 'first' for you, it is on the common list of complaints for all medical practitioners so march in and discuss it as though it's happening to someone else - you'll soon get over any initial embarrassment and within a few hours your vagina will probably be breathing a sigh of relief.

Banish Bacterial Vaginosis

A BV free vagina is a happy vagina. The bacteria in your vagina are capable of getting themselves back into balance so you can safely treat BV yourself with some of the home remedies mentioned previously. If a home remedy works for a short period but doesn't stop your BV from coming back, a prescribed cream or antibiotic pill may do the trick for you.

Be aware that antibiotics can be expensive and also harsh on your body (literal translation of the word 'antibiotic' means 'against life') so they will kill ALL bacteria, the bad guys *and* that resident family of good guys. Antibiotics can also fling open the door to yeast villains like thrush.

Antibiotics: - 77% of all women who treat BV with pharmaceutical antibiotics suffer from reoccurrence within months. If you prefer to use antibiotics, check for compatibility with any other meds/supplements that you take. Follow any instructions related to alcohol intake and also taking the prescribed antibiotic with food.

Some common antibiotics prescribed for BV include:

- Clindamycin (generic Cleocin)

- Tindemax

- Flagyl (don't drink alcohol while taking this or you could have nausea and vomiting)

Many of you have already discovered that these antibiotics don't work for you so it's time to seriously consider travelling down another road. As you trial various alternatives, use your pH test kit to monitor how your body responds then fine tune the treatment to *regain your acidic balance.*

Antibiotic Creams: - are about as effective as oral antibiotics but can weaken latex condoms and diaphragms (it's the STD's you're protecting yourself from, not the pregnancy, unless you're in perimenopause)

Intra Vaginal pessaries: - ask your doctor for a prescription or try lactobacillus acidophilus tablets orally and vaginally.

BV can be passed between female sexual partners - if you have no more symptoms after treatment you can be fairly sure that you've cleared up this condition. However, if you are prone to recurrences practice the recommendations listed on 'Reduce Your Risk of a Plumbing Problem' and if you still have multiple sex partners, keep your proven remedy on standby.

Vaginal Thrush – Not Had It? Lucky You!

Thrush is an overgrowth of the yeast cells that live naturally in your vagina - it is not a sexually transmitted disease. This overgrowth of yeast cells occurs when your vaginal pH is out of whack (you know it should be slightly acidic). Like bacterial vaginosis, thrush can also drive you nuts when it cries 'immunity!' but *unless you regain the pH balance in your vagina*, this intelligent little sucker won't succumb to antifungal and other traditional treatments.

Do not use any over the counter treatments for yeast infections until your thrush has been confirmed by a reliable test kit or a doctor. Different infections can have similar symptoms so you may mistakenly think you have a yeast infection when you actually have bacterial vaginosis, a UTI or genital herpes. You don't want to delay correct treatment as well as your recovery with a DIY misdiagnosis. I don't want to dash hopes here but doctors don't always beat this one either.

Symptoms of Thrush (Candida albicans, Monilia, Candidiasis)

- white discharge like cottage cheese with a yeasty smell

- itching/burning, perhaps a rash in your genital area

- swelling or redness of your vulva or vagina

- stinging feel during sex or when you pee

- tears/splits in the skin around your vagina

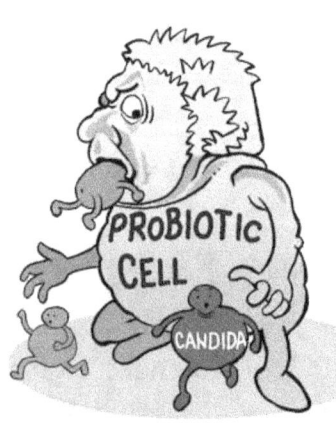

Treatment: you will be sick of reading this by now but the key to success is restoring your vaginal pH balance by gobbling up the yeast cells.

- if you want a good start to getting rid of thrush yourself, check out a proven winner, Threelac, a Probiotic containing *Enterococcus Faecalis* (not *Enterococcus Faecium*)

- popular anti-fungal and enzyme treatments like Monistat and Canestan give relief - some may clear up new or weak thrush infections, if you use pessaries, wear old knickers to bed for obvious reasons

Prevention: follow best practice in basic vaginal care (page 11) and also practice the good stuff on page 35.

Untreated Thrush Can Holiday Up North!

Did you know that if thrush gets well entrenched in your body it can end up in your mouth? Not nice. Now that you're in a position to detect the early signs of vaginal thrush, you'll be able to stop those feisty yeast cells from travelling North.

By 'travelling North', I mean that the yeast cells, which started off in your large intestine have multiplied and traveled up through your small intestine, multiplied their way on into your stomach and esophagus and have ended up in your mouth. Oral thrush causes a white coating on your tongue and inside your cheeks (a white coating on your tongue can indicate conditions other than oral thrush of course but a swab test will confirm these)

I can't find out where this test originated but it seems to be a fairly reliable and easy way of finding out if you have a well entrenched case of Candida.

The spit test - you'll probably never have to do it yourself but you never know when you may have reason to pass on this information, not the best pick up line but it could be useful trivia.

As soon as you wake in the morning work up as much saliva as you can and spit into a glass of water. Don't eat or drink anything or even brush your teeth before doing this. Yeast cells are heavier than your saliva cells so when you spit into a glass of water they will sink to the bottom, fascinating, albeit somewhat gross.

Floating saliva is healthy saliva = no yeast cells present

If your saliva sinks to the bottom (oh, oh) or is a speckled cloudy mass or has little tendrils hanging down, chances are you have Candida. It may take up to half an hour to see the results so be patient and wear your specs if need be.

Saliva test

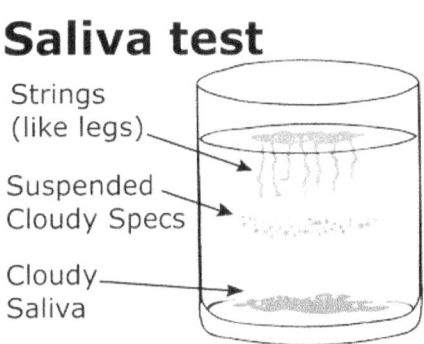

Strings (like legs)

Suspended Cloudy Specs

Cloudy Saliva

If the test is positive, grab some of that good probiotic with *Enterococcus Faecalis* (yeast cells cannot become immune to this probiotic, unlike some others) and fingers crossed, in a little while you'll be amazed at the results.

Plumbing Problems

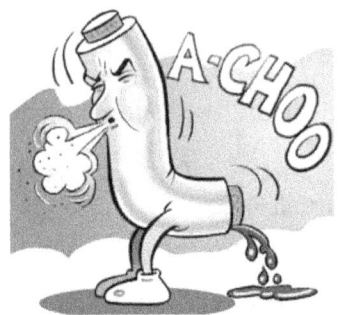

Joy of Joys, you clock up several decades of vagina mileage and now you have to change your knickers after a sneeze! Your purse is stocked with 'Poise' pads because you haven't been doing your Kegels, your bladder and pelvic floor are suffering collateral damage from 'ripening' and you're in line for an Oscar in incontinence. But wait….there's more! Plumbing problems caused by inflammation of the bladder and urethra are common occurrences for the over 40s.

Mellowing changes in your vagina, bladder and urethra* make you more susceptible to a urinary tract infection (UTI). Diabetes, stones or a tumor in your urinary tract, wearing a catheter or having a disease in your kidneys or bladder can also trigger a UTI. If you get a UTI every time you have intercourse it's because bothersome bacteria have been pushed up your vagina to your urethra.

E. Coli - most infections of the urinary tract are caused by one type of bacteria, *Escherichia coli* which normally lives in your colon yet happily goes 'walkabout'.

These symptoms are indicators that you may have a UTI:

- pain when you pee and you may even have a temperature

- wanting to pee very frequently or leaking urine – if you need to pee more than 6 times a day, this could indicate trouble

- feeling like you want to pee even though you've just been

- strong and unpleasant smelling pee that may be cloudy or bloody

- back pain, fever, chills, nausea and vomiting may occur if the infection has invaded your kidneys

Our female design doesn't help us – as a female of the species, one thing you can't change is the position and length of your urethra which was designed by a higher power to be located closer to your bum bacteria than a male's urethra is in relation to his bum bacteria. This short stroll from the back door to the front door means the bothersome bacteria have less distance to cover from one female orifice to another before paddling upstream to cause trouble.

A UTI is confirmed via a pee sample, which you can do yourself if you prefer, with a dip stick type test kit used on your first morning pee (about 90% reliable).

*the tube from your bladder that carries urine to your vagina

Reduce Your Risk of a Plumbing Problem

You may not be optimistic about getting back in the sexual saddle but if you're over 40 it's sensible to do what you can to prevent adding a UTI to your portfolio of maturity related problems. If you're sexually active, read this twice.

Here are some good things to do:

- we goddesses are notorious for 'holding it in' while we finish off a task, well don't, it's one of the worst things you can do to encourage bacteria to develop into a full blown infection (your bladder muscles eventually weaken and then don't empty out your pee efficiently, thus leaving bacteria to thrive)

- wipe from front to back after going to the toilet to stop bacteria from your bum doing the limbo across to your vagina and up your urethra

- enjoy 4 oz cranberry juice twice a day (see page on treatment of UTI's for 'no sugar' option or take 500IU of Vitamin C a day)

- wear cotton undies so moisture can escape and create a less favorable climate in which bacteria can breed

- pee before and after intercourse to flush bacteria down and out

- wash your genitals before and after sex to prevent transfer of bacteria (you can't see bacteria so wash even if you think you're clean)

- try varying your positions for intercourse to reduce friction on your urethra (you're never too old to try something new - use this medical reason as your excuse, it's not very romantic but it trumps the risk)

- take showers more often than baths – this helps to prevent those clever little breeders from sailing up river into your vagina and on into your urine canal

- drink warm water each morning with a capful of apple cider vinegar

You get an infection when bacteria from your digestive tract cling to the opening of the urethra and begin to multiply. Depending on how much you drink and eat, you pee around a quart and a half of urine every day. Normally, the flow of urine helps to wash any bacteria out of your body.

The little E. Coli brigade loves a route march and given the chance, will happily set off to cause trouble in your bladder and kidneys if you ignore a bladder infection.

Fix Your Plumbing Problems

Ok, so you've done all you can to lower your risk of getting a UTI but you've pulled the short straw anyway and you're darned uncomfortable. What can you do to get rid of it as soon as possible?

A course of antibiotics and/or pain relievers is the standard treatment which you'll be offered. While antibiotics have their place, I'd be asking about side effects if I were you and thoroughly exploring other options as well. You often end up needing several courses of antibiotics so choose your weapon wisely.

Below are some favorite alternatives to antibiotics for treating a UTI:

- take D-mannose once a day – a natural, safe, non toxic, dietary supplement which contains the active ingredient found in cranberries but does NOT contain high levels of fructose found in processed cranberry juice- this also works to prevent recurrence

- at the first sign of a UTI, take over the counter herbal remedies or extra doses of Vitamin C /500IU a day (check for compatibility with the pharmacist if you're taking other meds)

- drink warm water each morning with a capful of apple cider vinegar

- take cranberry pills every half hour till symptoms disappear

- cut down on milk, ice cream and milk drinks. not natural, unsweetened yoghurt though

- cut down on coffee, alcohol and citrus juices

- drink lots of water to dilute your pee and flush out bacteria

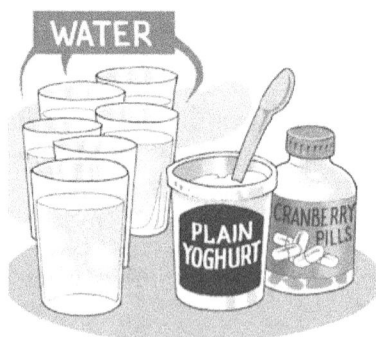

Vaginal Bleeding

Assuming you do not suffer from hemophilia or Willebrand disease and assuming that you have not had a period for years, bleeding after you reach 50 is a worry.

Vaginal bleeding may be caused by:

- damage to the thin and fragile walls of your vagina caused by intercourse

- cervical polyps or lesions on your genitals

- a vaginal infection

- cancer

Drugs: certain drugs can trigger vaginal bleeding so you need to get your doctor to find out if this is the case with you (e.g. Anti clotting drugs, Aspirin etc)

Elderly goddesses have the severest loss of estrogen and are at a higher risk of vaginal atrophy (there's that awful word again) which means that the walls of elderly vaginas are extremely thin and fragile and can bleed from the slightest damage. Even small tears open pathways to infection so don't ignore them.

A slight scratch or spot now and again is not what I mean by 'vaginal bleeding'. Bleeding that soaks a sanitary pad or is accompanied by any pain must be taken seriously.

Abnormal bleeding if you're elderly is a sign that something is wrong so please get a thorough investigation done to rule out a serious condition like cancer. For most of you, you'll probably find that the bleeding is associated with vaginitis, a UTI or some other less worrying condition, however, don't lose precious time in finding out because the sooner you confirm the cause of the bleeding, the better chance you have of successfully dealing with it.

Blood loss affects blood pressure - a severe drop in blood pressure could place you in a life or death situation. DO NOT try home remedies or over the counter medications for this one!

N.B. If you are still the owner of a uterus, cervix and a pair of ovaries and have significant bleeding, you need to get straight to the doctor to rule out any form of cancer or bladder problem.

Vaginal Warts = Unhappy Vagina

Just to be clear, warts in a vagina are not related to genital herpes (the herpes simplex2 virus) but to a common virus found on our skin and mucous membranes called the HPV or *human papillomavirus*, of which there are over 100 members in this club. The most common HPV types that infect the genital area are HPV types 6 and 11, which are benign (types 16 and 18 are found in cancers of the cervix). The benign guys, 6 and 11, set up abode in our genitals very easily. There is no cure for HPV but...

The good news is that the genital wart guys are a low risk type of genital HPV which usually go for younger women in their first years of sexual activity. If you are without symptoms, your immune system has probably clobbered any genital HPV you may have had.

The bad news is that for 40 plus women this unwanted bonus that comes with wild nights of adventurous passion can still be donated as a freebie to any ripe vagina that's back on the intimate dating scene.

How do warts sneak across the border? – warts sneak up on you when your private bits have skin to skin contact with someone else's private bits, not through bodily secretions or blood. Once the virus has become your squatter, genital HPV

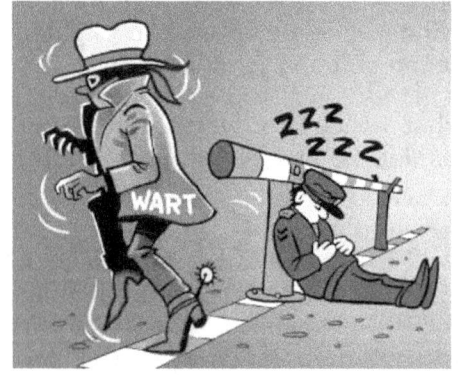

stays with you till your expiry date but don't stress, you can control it very well.

New sexual partners, even late in life, who carry genital HPV and gallantly roll on their condoms don't provide complete protection for you I'm afraid, because you could both join other exposed areas that are still infected and voila! There's no prize for guessing that you're at a lower risk of picking up these warty lodgers if you're not having sex. That's made your day, I'll bet.

Single or clustered warts come in a fashionable flesh or pink color, can be various shapes and sizes and usually take up to 3 months to develop after infection.

Warts are often only discovered by your doctor unless you can see them or suspect them to be the cause of itching, burning, bleeding or discharge. Symptoms are the same for everyone - they just appear in different places.

Vaginal Warts - Treatment

It helps to be lighthearted while resuscitating your ageing vagina but genital HPV and vaginal warts do cause emotional distress and embarrassment, especially if you get clobbered later in life. Add this to the smack in the face from menopausal challenges and it's hard to raise a smile. Genital HPV is very common, if you have it, it's likely that your current partner probably has it too. Hey, you need to know.

Topical control is the first line of approach - once genital HPV is diagnosed the tenacious little resident will lie dormant in your body forever, regardless of treatment. You or your partner may have had the virus for years without knowing so don't be too quick to dump the blame for your benign bumps.

Treatment will depend on the type, size and location of your warts and on what you're prepared to pay. Professional options include:

- freezing – cryosurgery, uses liquid nitrogen and has few side effects

- burning – electrocautery - not a blow torch but a low voltage electric probe or looped wire which is used under local anesthesia, hooray

- application of a chemical like TriChloroacetic acid which is also used for face peels but don't try this at home folks

- laser therapy – expensive, requires a longer healing time, I'd research this method more if I were you as it is being questioned over possibly destroying the local immune system

- interferon injections – a last resort if all other methods fail

Beware a drug called Aldara (active ingredient Imiquimod) if recommended for any type of application to 'boost your immune system to deal with this virus'. As prominent Gold Coast cancer specialist Dr Michael Tait says, "In my opinion, based on my observations and research, Aldara should be classified as a criminally dangerous material if used on any open or potentially open skin area." Imiquimod is on the National Cancer's list of hazardous chemicals and is a known carcinogen. Aldara affects your immune system- is yours strong enough to take a risk with this drug? Thoroughly research the risks of using this drug.

Warts can re appear after treatment so if you want to keep your vagina happy, ditch the ciggies, cut down the sugar and alcohol, keep stress levels low and keep your immune system as healthy as possible.

Sneaky Genital Herpes

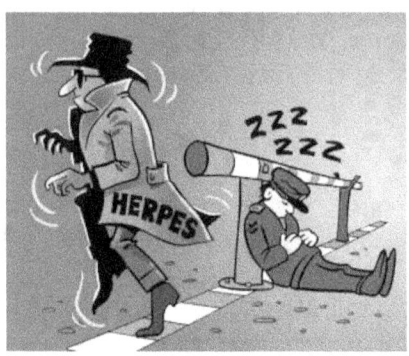

If you're about to have a new sexual encounter, *especially* if you've previously enjoyed a long term sexual relationship with one person, you are at risk of catching herpes. *Women are almost twice as likely to get genital herpes as men.*

Genital herpes is sexually transmitted and this little sucker of a virus will be your no.1 fan for life once he moves in. There is no cure for genital herpes but you can successfully curfew the little lodger and confine him to his room.

80% of people with genital herpes don't realize they have this travelling companion on board so passing it on is not an act of malicious intent. This clever little body hopper extends his family through all forms of skin to skin contact, especially during sex and regardless of your persuasion.

Facts about genital herpes - Herpes Simplex type 2 a relative of the common cold sore virus Herpes Simplex type 1.

- 20% people carry it without having symptoms

- you can pass it on without having symptoms

- you can have the virus for years without knowing it and without having symptoms, it 'hides' in your nerve root cells

- you only need *one* sexual encounter with a carrier to catch it (not fair!)

- there can be years between you getting herpes and the symptoms appearing (if at all)- your most recent sexual partner may not have passed it on to you so be careful whom you blame!

- 60% people don't realize their symptoms indicate genital herpes

- you can develop genital herpes if someone with cold sores treats you to oral sex

- the little blighter doesn't hop aboard in a spa, from a towel or a toilet seat

Unfortunately, ignorance is bliss - a test for genital herpes is not included in standard STD tests, if it was, maybe there wouldn't be so many ignorant carriers running around.

Genital Herpes - Symptoms

You own a vagina and a pair of labia, which, if they get blisters on them because of a blighter called Herpes Simplex2 - ouch! Get help for your poor vagina if she's suffering any of Herpy's symptoms below and do it before you let her have sex again. If you discover that Herpy's already moved in, you need to prevent his behavior from worsening and reduce his chances of moving in on your lover.

A blood test and a swab test from blisters or ulcers (best done within 3 days of a sore appearing) will reveal if Herpy has sneaked in when the game was playing. No, it's not fair. Herpy can knock you around emotionally at first. Throw a baked spud at the wall, swear at next door's cat and do whatever you need to do to get rid of your anger but don't let genital herpes control your life – the virus can be treated and managed very successfully.

Symptoms of genital herpes

- redness, tingling and itching around your vaginal area

- a rash or small cracks or splits in the skin

- the appearance of tiny sores which you could think are pimples or blisters and which are painful

- 'flu like symptoms at first as your immune system deals with the virus —a fever, headaches or pains in the your back and legs (subsequent outbreaks don't have these symptoms)

- a vaginal discharge that you may think is thrush and persists for 1 to 3 weeks (caused by one little gangster named Herpetic cervicitis)

Don't panic at the pictures - be aware that many text books and online images show photos of severe cases of herpes lesions. If genital herpes is neglected and complications set in, it can be so painful to pee that some women end up wearing a catheter as an unfashionable accessory (what!?) but in most cases, initial outbreaks of herpes are not worthy of horror screams and can be treated quickly.

Recurring attacks - you'll probably never know what triggers a new crop of your genital cold sores but it's likely to occur in the same spot as before.

Recurring attacks are not caused by re infection but by something (illness, sexual activity, stress, who knows?) that awakens the sleeping lodger to leave his room again. Fresh crops of genital herpes may not be as painful as the first, don't usually last as long, become less frequent with time and may eventually stop altogether. There ya go!

Genital Herpes – Prevention and Treatments

70% of carriers pass Herpy the hitch hiker around on viral shedding days when virus cells are left behind on a partner. Shedding occurs with and without visible symptoms. Early treatment is the key to success, either organically or with drugs.

Certified antiviral plant extracts in special organic essential oils and soap (H-Balm) neutralize and destroy Herpy's virus, help prevent recurring outbreaks and stop Herpy from penetrating into uninfected cells.

Antiviral drugs like aciclovir (*Zovirax*) and famciclovir (*Famvir*) stop Herpy from breeding, reduce the number and severity of his attacks, reduce viral shedding and slim down the chance of Herpy hitch hiking to another partner.

Preventative measures you should also take:

- use condoms, male or female ones, during sex - you won't get 100% protection because condoms can't cover *other* infected parts where viral shedding occurs but barriers are great 'bouncers' for your vagina venue

- wash your hands if you come into contact with a naked Herpy (herpes sores) particularly new blisters - Herpy can hitch-hike on your hands from site to site on your own body and then onto your partner

- avoid sexual contact involving your genitals until sores have gone

To make life more comfy:

- wear loose, cotton knickers and avoid tight jeans

- wrap an ice-cube in a face washer and hold it on the tingly bits for an hour (aagh, did I say 'comfy'!?) when you feel tingling but blisters haven't appeared, it may stop them from forming

- apply Betadine on your sores to keep them clean and dry

- take your preferred analgesic if you need pain relief

- use both hands to hold apart the lips of your vulva and stop urine from touching your blisters when you pee

- if it hurts to pee, pee in the bath (hey, whatever works) or pour warm water over the painful area as you pee

- use a blow dryer set on low or cool to dry your genitals after washing

- drink lots of water to dilute your pee and get more rest if you can

How to Live with Herpy the Lodger

As a despondent and outraged landlord, don't be shy in talking to other landlords about your Herpes lodger. I know you want to closet Herpy away, literally but there's no need to agonize in silence over this embarrassing problem. If you're having a hard time coping with the psychological shock, a genital herpes support group will give you the relief you need. Other sufferers will keep you up to date with the latest treatments and help you to get your feelings and your life back in balance.

By the way, if you're worried that genital herpes will lead to you getting cancer of your cervix don't be.

Once you get on top of your treatment regime and quickly pounce on an imminent outbreak, you'll find that life as you knew it pre herpes is back to normal. Be constantly on the alert for that tell tale tingling sign that Herpy is about to leave his room and have a tantrum and your cherished vagina will thank you.

Let your sexual partner know - once you're sure that Herpy's on board, always, always let your partner(s) know before you do any type of canoodling. This is the responsible thing to do and makes it much easier for both of you to reduce the chances of that little blighter smuggling his offspring across the border.

Tell your partner of your history with genital herpes and that there may be times when you can't have sex. If you are considerate of each other needs when it comes to using condoms and taking other precautions, you're relationship won't suffer any collateral damage.

It can be awkward at first, talking to your lover (especially a new senior one) about herpes but a frank and honest discussion is the best way to be respected and to arrive at an amicable way for both of you to have safe, worry free sex.

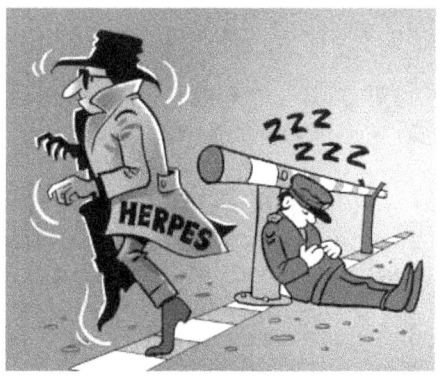

FC2 is the new female condom – try it at least once, your male partner may be delighted with your offer to use a female condom and in reducing condom friction in your vagina it may be more comfy for you too.

Be brave and speak up - if you aren't in a long term relationship you have every right to ask about your partner's sexual health history too.

Chlamydia Alert for the Over 40s

Previously, there's been a somewhat erroneous expectation of the post menopausal female of our species to be 'past it', sexually inactive or in a sexually safe monogamous relationship. With the emergence of the alleged Cougar, the popularity of on line dating services and the changing relationship norms of today's society, over 40s females need to be really savvy about managing the skin to skin aspects of their new intimate relationships.

Great, we may not need pregnancy protection any more girls but as well as protecting ourselves from gold digging gigolos looking for 'Mother with Benefits' we do need to protect ourselves from other unwelcome catches. Our mellowing vaginas are past the spring chicken stage which means that we are more susceptible to picking up a sexually transmitted infection (STI) or to missing the signs that we may already have one.

Any sexually active person can be infected with Chlamydia. (_Chlamydia trachomatis_) I thought it best to mention this little Charlie (you'll notice that I give the villains male names - don't read anything into that) because he is a very common bacterial STI which you probably think only infects the young ones. Incidences of middle aged goddesses getting lumbered with STI's are on the rise. . You'll be safe from future fetuses once you exit menopause but if you embark on new sexual journeys with new partners, please be a savvy, condom loaded gal and protect yourself and your vagina from STIs.

Symptoms of Chlamydia - are like those of a UTI (abnormal vaginal discharge or a burning sensation when urinating and crampy pain in the lower abdomen). Chlamydia can also cause conjunctivitis. BUT the real bummer is that _most women don't have any symptoms_ so Charlie Chlamydia romps wherever he pleases inside your body, free to hop happily onto someone else's if you give him half a chance.

Diagnosis - Chlamydia is diagnosed from a pap smear or from swabs you can take yourself. Chlamydia can't be diagnosed from a blood test.

Treatment is simple and effective though it can cause a few uncomfortable side effects such as diarrhea, nausea and abdominal pain however, just a single prescribed dose of antibiotics - Azithromycin (Zithromax) or the less costly Doxycycline (Vibramycin, Oracea, Adoxa, Atridox) usually sends Charlie packing. Don't have sex until at least a week after treatment. If your partner is receiving treatment for Chlamydia, don't have sex until at least a week after _both_ of you have been treated.

Stop Charlie entering your door simply by using a condom (male or female variety) and don't have unprotected sex with a new partner unless you're sure that they have passed their STD exam!

Prolapses – What Are They?

Genital prolapses have a lot in common with hernias. Both are due to weakness of supporting tissues. A vaginal prolapse means you've got a case of saggies in your pelvic floor darling. Your over-stretched ligaments are no longer strong enough to prevent gravity from dragging the pelvic organs surrounding your vagina south. Your bladder, urethra, uterus, small bowel and rectum can cause bother in vaginaville. It's nice to relax as one mellows but this is really going *too* far. A severe prolapse is distressing and can have a significant impact on your daily life - a mild one is hardly noticeable.

The big 'M', estrogen loss and childbirth contribute to prolapse potential but there are other factors that can result in this vaginal misery, including previous pelvic surgery, a tumor in your pelvis or very rarely, a uterus enlarged by fibroids.

A vaginal vault prolapse can occur after a hysterectomy (fix one thing and cause another, not fair) Without a uterus, there is no longer a decent support structure at the top of your vagina which then droops poor little thing, putting extra stress on your already over stretched ligaments which in turn aren't strong enough to stop her from falling towards the door.

A uterine prolapse occurs when your cervix and uterus drop down towards your vaginal entrance. Happy Days.

A bowel, bladder or urethra prolapse occurs when your rectum, urethra or bladder drops down and pushes into the wall of your vagina. You may get the perks of incontinence or constipation with this one too and if you're unlucky, you'll pee during sex! Great. We gals get more than our fair share of whammies don't we?

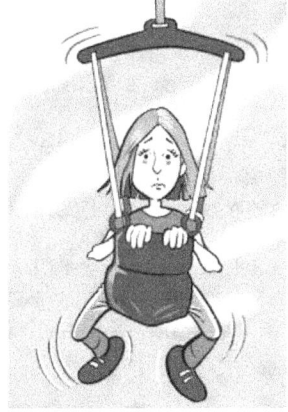

Life's not fair, God. I want my happy vagina back.

Vaginal Prolapse – Signs and Symptoms

Symptoms of a prolapse differ depending on which organ is 'droopy' and how far or in which direction it has drooped. It's hard to keep up with your daily activities if you suspect that something is falling down in your lady garden, especially if you're struggling with uncomfortable symptoms. Your doctor will tell you whether or not you have this problem and you'll soon be on your way to a successful vagina recovery.

You may not have any symptoms for a mild prolapse but an early warning sign that you should watch out for is slackness in the walls of your vagina. Prolapses are graded 1-4 or according to their degree of severity and each type can have its own set of variations.

I won't detail each type of medical prolapse and its associated symptoms here, but to help you with a self check in order to begin a conversation with your doctor, this check list below will give you an idea of what to look out for with a prolapse that's more advanced.

Some common symptoms include:

- constipation that occurs frequently

- a large lump at the entrance to your vagina

- pain during intercourse

- frequent urinary tract infections (UTIs)

- a dragging feeling, heaviness or pain in your abdomen or lower back or a feeling that 'something is falling down' especially when sneezing or coughing or after standing for a long time

- leakage of urine or even feces when you cough, sneeze or change position (don't immediately think prolapse with a slight pee sneeze alone, this is a common over 40s problem)

- incomplete emptying of either your bladder or bowel

- pain in your lower back - a dull ache that won't go away

Seek help sooner rather later, upgrade your medical insurance if you have to - your health and sanity from here on in are your main essentials in life.

Prolapse - Tips to Prevent

I hope that you aren't suffering from a serious vaginal problem and that you bought this book for vaginal health 'insurance' - you may even be one of those goody goodies who does her daily Kegels. As your vagina heads towards 50, 60 and 70 years of age, she merits special attention to help her to avoid the miseries of a prolapse and happily jig on to her 80th and 90th birthdays.

Prolapse is a real threat to older vaginas – here are a few tips which will help you to avoid one in the first place:

- contract your pelvic floor muscles whenever you can - that means when you sneeze, cough, laugh or blow your nose (traffic light 'quickies' won't cut it girls). Persevere, strengthening muscles takes months, instructions for Kegel exercises page 13

- try to maintain a recommended weight for your height (easier said than done, I agree)

- a single action of straining can cause a prolapse so avoid constipation by whatever method you prefer

- never strain to empty your bowels when sitting - your colon is unsupported and you have a kink at your anus so 'pushing downwards' literally forces your pelvic floor downwards

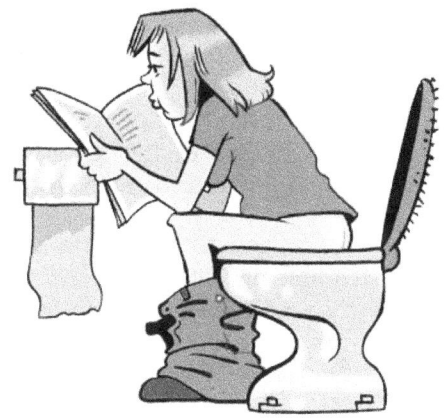

- practice being the Queen - avoid heavy lifting, including frequent lifting of grandchildren and Corgis

- sit down regularly to counter gravity if you have to stand for long periods, think of your vagina struggling to hold up the world 'down under'

- go power walking rather than running or start a 'non-jiggling' type of dancing class, you never know what other fringe benefits might come your way!

- seek personalized physiotherapy exercises – especially if you already have early signs of a prolapse - you'll even learn how to poo in the correct position ('What?' Yeay, there's an accomplishment to brag about!)

Vaginal Prolapse - Treatments

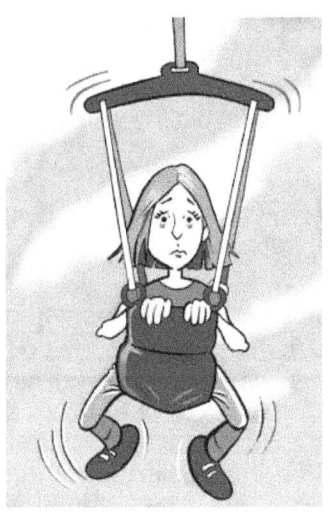

Please don't put off a visit to your doctor if you suspect that you may have a prolapse, it will get worse until you treat it. Early warning of a prolapse is slackness in the walls of your vagina so be vigilant with the symptoms I've mentioned previously.

Once the 'saggy' has been professionally identified, appropriate treatment will be explained for your specific type of prolapse. Be careful about comparing notes if you have a prolapse pal - your friend could have a completely different type of saggy problem to yours that requires different treatment (my grandma, God rest her soul, seemed quite disappointed when she didn't get a colostomy bag following colon cancer surgery like her friend did!)

These are the most common options for treating a prolapse:

- pelvic floor exercises (doh!) with or without the help of a professional

- estrogen replacement therapy – ask your doctor if this is appropriate

- bio feedback – via electrical stimulation - calm down, it's not torture and it's not used to treat prolapses as much nowadays. Basically, a sensor is attached to your vagina to help you to find out which muscles to squeeze and for how long

- pessaries to keep the prolapse in place – a pessary is a flexible ring made of rubber which is fitted into your vagina to hold up the walls. A pessary may be worn for a long 'scaffolding job' or used as a temporary measure to relieve symptoms and incontinence prior to surgery (remove it before sex, if that's still on your to do list)

- surgery is usually effective and will correct all weaknesses at the same time since one prolapse often means another is likely to develop (two for one, a bargain). Expect 2-4 days in hospital or only overnight with robot assisted surgery

Depending on the severity of your prolapse, you may not need surgery – you maybe able to treat it yourself with a plan from a physiotherapist. Chin up.

Electrical Stimulation for a Happy Vagina

No, it's not what you're thinking (but that will make your vagina happy too!) Biofeedback via electrical stimulation is a technique that helps people to use signals from their own bodies to treat a health issue. Biofeedback is used for all sorts of disorders including helping stroke victims to regain the use of their inactive muscles and as therapy for some athletes.

Bio feedback is not often used these days to treat a vaginal prolapse , however your doctor may mention it as a last resort to try to avoid surgery. Around one in eleven women will need surgery for a prolapse so smile smugly if you don't.

Caution: - Biofeedback therapy is not advised for persons with severe psychosis, depression or obsessional neurosis. It is dangerous for diabetics and people with endocrine disorders as it can change the need for insulin and other medications. *Please check with your doctor to see whether this is an appropriate treatment for you.*

There are a couple of bio feedback methods:

Option one: don't get squeamish when I tell you that the first option involves an electric probe that is applied to certain muscles on your pelvic floor or in your vagina. A measuring device connected to the probe controls the amount of current so you're not about to be deep fried! The procedure is painless. You'll feel a slight buzzing sensation and a contraction of your vaginal muscles.

The strength of this simulated squeeze is monitored and can be seen on a screen so you know how well (or not) your muscles are doing with each contraction.

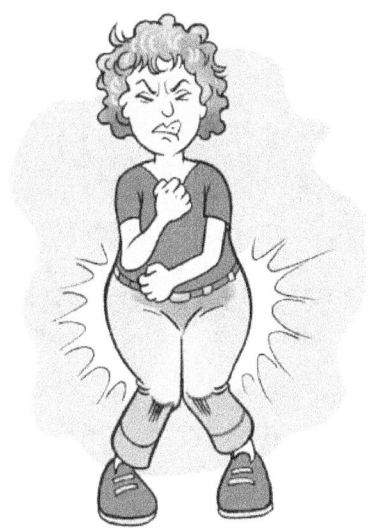

After a few contractions, you should be able to duplicate the squeezing/strengthening exercises yourself. Thereafter, DIY is always preferable to a probe job...and cheaper. Go Kegel Girl!

Option two: the second option for stimulating and strengthening the vaginal muscles is an electrical device that is not as intrusive as the probe, this device works by magnetically stimulating the pudendal nerve from outside the body. The pudendal nerve is seated deep in the pelvic regions of both males and females and is responsible for the functions and control of orgasms as well as urination and defecation. Lovely, that's one for the latte circle next time you meet.

Designer Vaginas

If your vagina could speak for herself she'd shout 'Back off!' to a knife wielding surgeon. Personally, I am not ashamed of my vulva and if a partner judges me on the appearance of my 'jewels down below' well, there's another problem to solve and it isn't a cosmetic one. I'm including this page FYI only because resculpting of 'lady lips' is gaining popularity. The perfect vagina does not exist, it is a creation of censorship rules for men's magazines in which the models genitals are digitally retouched. In my opinion, anyone who is considering labia surgery should be doing it for medical reasons only and then after serious consultation.

Shrinkage of the labia minora usually occurs naturally 'at our age' anyway but many women are distressed if these lips protrude outside their labia majora (the size of medically *'normal'* labia minora ranges from 2cm-10cm). Saggy and flappy labia cause so much mental anguish to some women that they are driven to letting a surgeon slice off bits of their labia in order to feel good about their bodies. Enlightened society? I wonder.

Cosmetic options for vagina rejuvenation - previously performed for fixing medical problems such as prolapses and stress urinary incontinence, are now carried out for appearance alone - such cosmetic procedures include:

Vaginoplasty: your vaginal opening is made narrower and your vagina is also tightened by cutting the muscles and reattaching them. Ouch.

Labiaplasty: excess flesh is cut off your protruding inner labial lips to 'tidy them up' and achieve symmetry.

Vaginal Liposuction: fat is relocated from your upper thigh or lower abdomen by liposuction then injected into your labia to make them look soft and plump.

Vulvar Lipoplasty: if you have too much fat on your mons pubis or outer labia (not likely in women our age) then surprise, surprise, you can have it removed.

Clitoral Hood Reduction: skin around the clitoris is trimmed off. NB. This procedure can reduce sensitivity. The hood often shrinks back after 40 anyway.

Experience counts – if you do opt for surgery on your vulva, ask a surgeon whose done LOTS of these procedures to explain in detail how this type of surgery will alter your body. Investigate the risks of scarring, infection and nerve damage.

Ask former clients how the procedures have affected their sex lives. If your goal is better sex, self confidence is a big factor in achieving this. There are ways of improving *sex confidence* by less drastic means – yes, even when you're over 40!

Your G-spot, A-spot AND U-spot - WHAT?!

Correct. The infamous and elusive G-spot is only one of FOUR sexual hot spots in your body. Don't fret, you won't fail the test if you don't find them all or can't get pleasure from doing a stint of work experience with them.

Your 4 sexual 'hot spots' – are your G-spot, A-spot, clitoris-and U spot. You don't lose brownie points for doubting that your G-spot exists because a) you don't know where yours is and b) if you have one, it's never swept you away with its orgasmic delights. Rejoice. Every woman has a G-spot and here's how to track yours down in case you're interested in finding out what all the fuss is about.

Your G-spot or 'Goddess Spot' is highly sensitive and is more of a *zone* or patch than a spot. It is on the FRONT, inside wall of your vagina about 2-3 inches in (5-8cm). You may need to put in some patient exploration to find it but it's definitely there and feels a bit 'spongy'. The missionary position did little to kick start this erogenous zone so it's no wonder the poor old Goddess Spot was ignored for so long- no one knew she was there! When you are aroused, erectile tissue surrounding your urethra swells, causing a small area of your vaginal wall to protrude out into your vagina – this is the G-spot. Not all women respond ecstatically to their G-spot being stimulated so relax, it's OK if yours doesn't.

G-spot injection - I'm not kidding, some women are having collagen injected into their G spot zone to enhance it in an attempt to increase sensitivity and give them better orgasms. The collagen used is similar to the substance used to plump up lips. Personally, I'll pass … on both.

Your A-spot (AFE-zone or Anterior Fornix Erogenous Zone) - just as the clitoris is the female equivalent of the male penis, the A-spot is the equivalent of the male prostate and is another of your hot spots. Your A-spot lies just above your cervix, at the innermost point of your vagina, between your cervix and your bladder. It's my understanding that direct stimulation of this spot produces violent orgasmic contractions (I can't confirm firsthand that it does but you can buy a special AFE vibrator to stimulate this zone). Your A-spot is not supposed to suffer from post-orgasmic over-sensitivity as your clitoris may.

Your U-Spot – this is another *zone* of sensitive, erectile tissue. Your U-spot lies just above and on either side of your urethral opening. Researchers have found that if this region is gently caressed, with the finger, the tongue, or the tip of the penis, there can be a powerful erotic response. Well, there you have it. You'll get plenty of free lattes if you tell your friends that they've got more than one hot spot and that YOU know where they are!

A Happy Vagina Tastes Good

Your vaginal juice is unique to you and could be slightly tangy or salty to taste, depending on what you eat and what meds or vitamin supplements you're on.

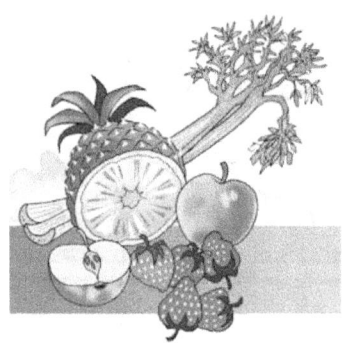

Lovers love vaginal juice. Lactobacilli, the same bacteria found in yogurt, are the resident good guy bacteria in your vagina. Healthy vaginal juice is variously described by lovers as tasting slightly sweet, slightly edgy, a bit like plain yogurt, slightly metallic, like a potato, a melon and slightly astringent which seems reasonable, given its acidic leaning.

Just because you're over 40 doesn't mean that you can't experiment with your juices (and your lover)

If your veteran vagina likes to be savored during sex, here are some gourmet tips to enhance your partner's tasty treat...

- keep 'her' clean – wash her exterior with non perfumed soap and water and remember that 'her indoors' is self cleaning

- hand your partner a glass of mouth wash before the froth and frolic

- gorge on fruits, especially pineapple and yoghurt (non sweetened variety) these favor a very happy and delicious tasting vagina

- seduction is all the sweeter for a feast of strawberries or apples

- celery also gives your vagina a sweet smell and taste

- go easy on the broccoli and asparagus pre passionate sessions – these veggies give a strong smell and taste to your vagina

- drinking beer will produce a bitter tasting vagina

- avoid smoking cigarettes – one can only imagine what that tastes like!

- be sensitive to your lover's needs – your 'taste' will vary from day to day so be receptive to feedback, especially on those slightly 'off' days

"Sex and golf are the two things you can enjoy even if you're not good at them"... Kevin Costner, Tin Cup.

Partner Page - Tips for Romeo

Spare a thought for the fact that men's testosterone supply also decreases as they age. While they're on the receiving end of your menopausal fall out, they may be struggling to come to terms with their own mellow cocktail of tiredness, depression and sexual problems. Poor darlings, we all know how 'men colds' are far worse than any woman's so BE KIND. Now is the time to dial up that sense of humor and

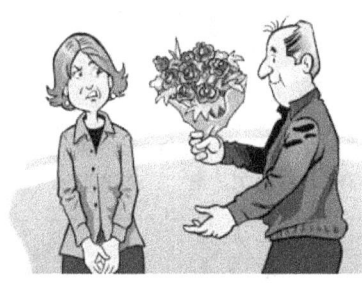

face the post meno music with a resounding chorus of 'We shall overcome!'

Sex is whatever 'sex' means to you - there are no rules for consensual loving and your trusty vagina may or may not join the party. A whispered endearment, a quick cuddle in the kitchen or a sensual feely session after the bedtime cocoa may be all that's desired for you and Romeo to arrive at a sexual truce, if not...

These tips may help your forgivably frustrated lover to understand your vagina's changing moods and their associated mental mysteries:

- if you've gone off sex, explain the strike in the hormone factory and tell him he's part of your renovation plans. Talk about your vaginal changes as lightheartedly as you can and involve him in the 'facelift' job – hey, experimentation could be your salvation along with blood pressure meds!!

- take a deep breath and suggest he buys you (both) a new self help 'toy'

- recreate special, feel good moments – go out, do something he loves that's not 'senior' focused

- a new relationship later in life can be daunting, especially if you've lost a long term partner – show your new Romeo that you feel good about your body(don't laugh) have fun and talk about your sexual 'diet'

- stress that time out for yourself is mandatory for your sanity and well being (preferably with loads of pampering) encourage him to do likewise

- if you're totally vaginally challenged, get professional help - a couple of sessions together will help your partner to understand your sexual distress and both of you to understand your new sex 'era'

- **Tornado Alert!** - leave silly 'emotional weather warning' stickers on the bathroom mirror so he can run for cover and rally to your rescue with roses on those unpredictable stay-well-clear days

Sensual Strains for Silly Seniors

"You don't stop dancing because you grow old you grow old because you stop dancing."...Author Unknown

A little abandon in the privacy of your own home can be the best vaginal therapy ever if you're game enough to fan the flames of seduction with a candlelit dance session for your beloved. Self - conscious? Remove your beloved's glasses first!

It's never too late to turn the music down low, lock the dog in the laundry and get into that sexy lingerie (oh, alright then, the cotton nightie) and sashay around the bedroom. Your partner will think you've lost it completely but it's unlikely your efforts will be totally wasted. A few gyrations across the room to the strains of 'The Ultimate Bolero' can lead to some sensual cuddles and a good night's sleep (that's *all* you want, right?)

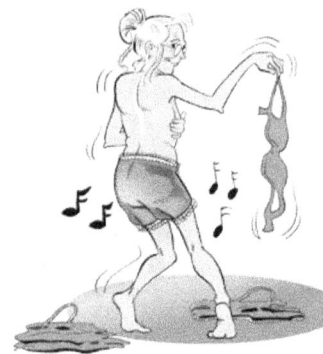

No partner? No excuse. Treat yourself to some sexy lingerie (or a new nightie) and dance anyway. If you're single again and on an E-Harmony date, timing is everything or you risk a bolt out the door before you can say 'Deep Heat Rub' - on the other hand, this could clinch the deal. Either way, take it slowly and think slinky, a little practice will soon get the blood flowing to your pink bits.

If you dare:

- Erotic Moods: The Collection, Vol. 1-3

- Erotic lounge Vol.1 (various artists)

- You Can Leave Your Hat On - Joe Cocker

- Music To Make Love By (various artists)

- Ravel's Greatest Hit: The Ultimate Bolero (plenty of Bolero versions to suit everyone)

- The stripper (arranged for organ) Tom Hazelton (Pipes of the Mighty Wurlitzer) includes lots of organ nostalgia for the 'well over 40's'

- Enigma: Love, Sensuality, Devotion (LSD) – not really stripper music but very erotic

...and remember-humor conquers all

Spoil Your Way to a Happy Vagina

Your vagina loves it when you are happy (recall those wonderful juices she squeezed out when you were *really, really* happy?). You don't need a partner or an excuse to find feel good ways to spoil yourself. Give yourself permission to consciously find at least one good thing a day, however small, that will give you a happy surge.

Don't leave your vulva and vagina out of your beauty routine. Your vagina is a special part of you that deserves daily consideration, if she's comfy and exhilarated from time to time, she'll age gracefully and happily. When you moisturize your face, moisturize your vulva and your vagina, after a manicure, moisturize your vagina, when you get back from the hairdresser's, trim your pubes, after your shower, moisturize your vagina. Got it? Embrace your authentic YOU, heritage monument and all.

Don't let other stuff, stuff you up - work, household chores, babysitting, volunteering, caring for aged parents and other time consuming activities can get in the way of 'ME time'. We all know what it's like to arrive at Sunday night and wonder where the heck the week went. You and your vagina need some SPACE.

Make up your own list of Virginia Woolf 'essentials' such as:

- quadruple ME time

- save for a pamper weekend or if that's a stretch (sorry, bad choice of words) a lovely aromatherapy massage will satisfy your skin contact needs

- join a fitness swim class or gym – and *go*, if only for a latte with the girls afterwards, if you didn't inherit the exercise gene, meet for a latte anyway

- read 'feel good' novels or watch 'feel good' movies, strawberries to hand

- buy a season ticket to the theatre , ballet, opera or sports club

- splurge on some ridiculously sexy lingerie – a 'Looks great!', fabulous bra and *matching* knickers can do wonders for a vagina's morale

- meditate, walk the beach or find your 'S spot' (solitude spot) I had a 'gin and tonic bench' in my garden which was a no go zone for everyone else...worked a treat

BUT don't give up on your Kegels - your vagina *adores* them!

A Final Word of Happiness...

As a goddess who chooses to cherish rather than admonish her mellowing pink bits, I wrote this guide to encourage you to honor your body in every aspect of its uniqueness and loveliness. There may be times when you wish you could swap parts with someone else but it's what's **inside** that really counts.

Keep in touch with your inner beauty – this never ages. Consider the young people of today who are bombarded by the media into believing that body image is everything. Anxieties and superficiality take some overcoming. You and I know that the 'beauty of youth' is rightly transient. What does ageing really mean to you? Be grateful and pass on your wisdom. It's up to us to showcase the grace and positives that maturity brings so that when it comes to leading the way and empowering the young, we can say 'I'm *OK*' and speak the truth.

Your body, like a much loved overcoat, may be looking a bit worn by now but as it ages, prepare yourself for the changes. Appreciate how well your body has served you and kept you going even under duress. I ask you to do one simple thing.

Next time you shower – smile at your sags and bags:

Lather up some fragrant frothing gel and slowly acknowledge every bit of your body, lovingly caressing every part of yourself that usually gets taken for granted in the morning's rub, scrub and grab the towel routine. Luxuriate in the perfumed foaming and give your senses a leisurely, indulgent treat.

- if your breasts are droopy, gently stroke them and ponder on the pleasure and nurturing they have given- to your children and your lovers

- if your belly is not as flat as it used to be, think of the womb within (maybe long gone) that may have been the safe nesting place for another life

- thank your legs for bearing your weight mile after exhausting mile..be grateful for this amazing system of yours... got the idea? Keep going.

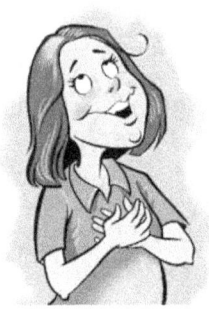 **Someone loves you for who you are**, warts and all (even if they happened to be covered in fur!) so embrace it and enjoy. Good luck with your resuscitation, happy pampering, wholesome healing, sumptuous loving and failing all else hold this thought:

"It's sad to grow old but nice to ripen"... Brigitte Bardot

Think Pink, Think Plump and Think Juicy

Further Sources

I have supported the information in this guide with personal research, input from generous women, product information and personal consultation with practicing health care providers.

For you online surfies, here are a few sites where you'll find further female facts: *information:*

www.nhs.uk

www.fwhc.org

www.about.com

www.mydr.com.au

www.cdc.gov/nchhstp

www.medicinenet.com

www.health.harvard.edu

www.womenshealth.gov

http://jama.ama-assn.org

www.mshc.org.au - Melbourne Sexual Health Centre

www.bashh.org - The British Association for Sexual Health and HIV Web site

www.myhormones.cc/bio-identical-hormones.html - Dr. Graeme Williams

www.womentowomen.com - Marcelle Pick OB/GYN, NP & Marcy Holmes, NP, Certified Menopause Clinician

www.susunweed.com - Susun Weed, author of women's health books, contributor to the Routledge International Encyclopedia of Women's Studies.

A huge pink, plump and juicy thank you to my talented illustrator, Vernon Knight, not only the fastest cartoonist in the West but now a much informed one!